Management of Diabetic Retinopathy

Management of Diabetic Retinopathy

AMP Hamilton
Consultant Surgeon, Moorfields Eye Hospital,
London, UK

MW Ulbig
Senior Registrar, Eye Clinic, Ludwig Maximilians
University, Munich, Germany

P Polkinghorne
Consultant Ophthalmologist and Vitreoretinal Surgeon to
Auckland Healthcare, New Zealand

BMJ
Publishing
Group

First published 1996
by the BMJ Publishing Group, BMA House, Tavistock Square,
London WC1H 9JR

British Library Cataloguing in Publication Data

A catalogue record for this book is available
from the British Library

ISBN 0 7279 0919 3

Typeset by Latimer Trend & Company Ltd, Plymouth
Printed by Craft Print, Singapore

Contents

Acknowledgments

The authors would like to thank the following people: Professor John Marshall and Professor Alec Garner for permission to use their slides; Jane Fallowes for her drawings; Mr KS Sehmi for his photographic advice and assistance; Professor Veit-Peter Gabel of the University Eye Hospital, Regensburg, Germany; and Mrs Lesley Gibons for her secretarial help.

Preface

This book aims to give a detailed account of the management of diabetic retinopathy; in fact this is predominantly laser therapy. It is disappointing that, after a period of more than 25 years of photocoagulation, this destructive mode of treatment is still the only effective therapy available for diabetic retinopathy, although there is evidence from the Oslo Study and the Diabetes Control and Complications Trial (DCCT) that improved control of diabetes mellitus may delay the development of diabetic retinopathy. Photocoagulation has, however, progressed to an extent where blindness can be prevented in most patients.

Over the years, there has been both advancing laser technology and the evolution of successful treatment regimens as a result of careful and exhaustive clinical trials. With the results from the Diabetic Retinopathy Study (DRS) and the Early Treatment Diabetic Retinopathy Study (ETDRS), the American Academy of Ophthalmology has introduced a programme named "Diabetes 2000" with the goal to prevent blindness from diabetic retinopathy by the year 2000. In Europe the WHO and the "St Vincent Declaration" aim at reducing the rate of blindness from diabetes by one third within five years. Moreover, the greater prevalence, longevity, and procreativity of diabetic individuals stress the importance of improving the ocular management of these patients. The establishment of specialist treatment centres is well advanced, but this experience in management must be extended further.

This book is designed to be a simple guide for use in the management of all the various aspects of diabetic eye disease.

PREFACE

Clearly, this book cannot be comprehensive and lacks extensive bibliography, but it suggests additional reading. With time, some of the techniques described in this book may evolve further with expanding knowledge and experience. The authors of this book are convinced that the most successful employment of lasers in retinal photocoagulation requires basic understanding of the technical detail of lasers and their mechanism of action within the retina. Thus, a chapter on lasers, their mechanisms of action, non-therapeutic side effects, and complications follows the chapter that introduces diabetic retinopathy.

Almost all definitions and treatment regimens recommended are consistent with the renowned studies of the DRS and ETDRS groups. Epidemiological data suggest that the type of diabetes mellitus, whether juvenile or maturity onset, insulin dependent or not, must also have an influence on indications for retinal photocoagulation. Thus, there is a special emphasis on this aspect, reflecting the latest treatment guidelines provided by the American Academy of Ophthalmology as well as the vast experience of this book's first author.

Primarily, this book is not designed for the shelf but rather for the white coat pocket, and this may explain why there is no comprehensive chapter on the pathogenesis of diabetic retinopathy, revealing all the knowledge and hypotheses on biochemical, endocrinological, and haemodynamic processes in diabetic eye disease. Instead there is major emphasis on the recognition of the various diabetic fundus lesions and their implications for photocoagulation treatment.

AMP Hamilton, MW Ulbig,
and P Polkinghorne
January 1996

viii

1 Diabetic retinopathy

Epidemiology

Diabetes mellitus is the major systemic cause of blindness in the Western World. It is also the leading cause of blindness in people of working age in these countries. In the United Kingdom diabetic eye disease results in about 1000 registered blind patients per year. In total, 2% of the British diabetic population are blind (8000–10 000 people in the United Kingdom) accounting for 7–8% of all blind registrations. A diabetic person is 10–20 times more likely to go blind than a non-diabetic person and indeed diabetes is the most common cause of blindness in the 30–60 year age group. Of the registered blind diabetic people 44% are over the age of 70 and 92% are over the age of 50; 75% are women. These data suggest that the most common blind diabetic person in the United Kingdom is a type II diabetic woman. The major risk factor for blindness in these patients is diabetic macular oedema. Thus the importance of focal and grid photocoagulation for diabetic maculopathy is emphasised. Also the indication for panretinal treatment in these patients, which can cause macular oedema to deteriorate, should be made carefully. The rising incidence of blind diabetic people, in spite of improved photocoagulation techniques, is the result of the increased longevity and procreativity of the population, and a relative inability to prevent late vascular complications.

The natural history and risk factors in diabetic retinopathy

Any studies of the natural history of diabetic retinopathy are marred by the fact that effective photocoagulation treatment is now established and that the guidelines for when to start treatment and the techniques of treatment are well documented. The study of the natural history of diabetic retinopathy is also difficult because of the variability of the disease, and the numerous factors that may influence its course and outcome. The natural history of diabetic retinopathy can be assessed in terms of type of diabetes mellitus, change in retinopathy appearance, and the chances of going blind.

Type of diabetes mellitus

In terms of type of diabetes mellitus, those with type I diabetes have predominantly proliferative diabetic retinopathy, and those with type II tend to have macular oedema. Kohner found that 50% of those with proliferative retinopathy had an onset of diabetes mellitus before the age of 20 years, whereas 75% of those with diabetic macular oedema had the onset of diabetes after the age of 40.

Change in retinopathy appearance and prognostic lesions

Fifty eight per cent of patients with mild non-proliferative retinopathy remain unchanged after four years of follow up, whereas 42% have progressed. Thirty five per cent of patients with severe non-proliferative diabetic retinopathy remain unchanged within the same period of time, but 65% have progressed, and 14% of these develop proliferative retinopathy. The presence of intraretinal microvascular abnormalities (IRMA) and the amount of intraretinal blotch haemorrhage are the best indicators for the progression of severe non-proliferative retinopathy and the development of

2

proliferation. Once macular oedema is present, then with time increase in oedema will inevitably occur. This is associated with further loss of visual acuity. The prognostic value of cotton wool spots for the progression of diabetic retinopathy has been overestimated previously, and no longer plays a major role. Cotton wool spots may, however, indicate associated arterial hypertension.

Chances of going blind

The chances of going blind within five years are shown in table 1.1, depending on age and retinal changes. It clearly demonstrates that the risk of going blind increases with age and the severity of retinal changes.

Table 1.1 Chances of going blind within five years from diabetic retinopathy

Age (years)	Fundus lesion	Percentage of blind patients
<29	Retinal microaneurysms	0
	Intraretinal haemorrhages + hard exudates	4
30–59	Retinal microaneurysms	12
	Intraretinal haemorrhages + hard exudates	24

Factors influencing the natural history of diabetic retinopathy

In those studies available about the natural history of diabetic retinopathy, there is a failure to identify factors other than those mentioned above, which may modify the outcome and the effect of photocoagulation treatment. These other factors can be further subdivided into external factors, internal factors, and ocular factors.

External factors

The external factors that may interfere with the course of diabetic retinopathy are diabetic control and diet, alcohol

3

consumption, smoking cigarettes, the contraceptive pill, and aspirin.

Control of diabetes mellitus A considerable amount has been published on the effect of improved quality of blood glucose contol on diabetic retinopathy. Early reports such as the KROC Study showed initial rapid deterioration of

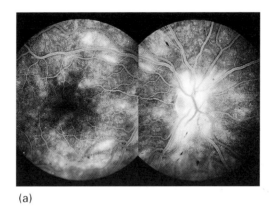

(a)

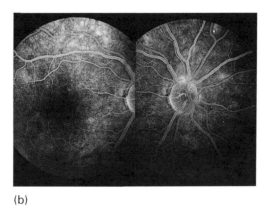

(b)

Figure 1.1 (a) Fluorescein angiogram of a poorly controlled diabetic patient, with capillary dilatations and microaneurysms. There is no real evidence of any capillary closure. (b) Fluorescein angiogram taken three months later, following institution of good control, showing the effect of the leaking capillaries

Table 1.2 Oslo Study: severity of diabetic retinopathy at baseline and after seven years in patients grouped according to mean blood glucose concentrations (HbA$_1$)

HbA$_1$ (%)	<9	9·1–10	>10
Mean number of retinal microaneurysms and haemorrhages			
At baseline	11·8	24·7	17·6
After 7 years	25·5	41·1	80·5
Change	+13·8	+16·4	+62·8

Box A   The influence of good and poor control on the development of diabetic retinopathy in dogs

Engerman's dogs
First 30 months of poor control
Followed by 30 months of good control = retinopathy

First 30 months of poor control
Followed by 30 months of poor control = retinopathy

First 30 months of good control
Followed by 30 months of poor control
   = *no* retinopathy

---

diabetic retinopathy associated with rapid improvement in blood glucose concentrations (fig 1.1). More recently, however, the beneficial effect of better long term control has been probed by the Diabetes Control and Complications Trial (DCCT) and the Oslo Study (table 1.2). Both studies assessed the severity of retinopathy at baseline and after seven years in patients grouped according to mean blood glucose concentrations measured as HbA$_1$.

There seems to be a point of no return once more severe diabetic retinopathy has become established. In the presence of large midperipheral areas of non-perfused retina, even perfect normoglycaemia, as achieved by pancreatic transplanation, is unable to prevent the formation of proliferative diabetic retinopathy. The Engerman dog studies (box

5

A) have shown that good control of blood glucose concentration is important with the onset of the disease.

The Oslo Study and the DCCT, however, come to the conclusion that even secondary intervention by long term lowering of glycated haemoglobin has a beneficial impact on non-proliferative diabetic retinopathy.

b *Alcohol consumption* There is a controversy about the influence of drinking habits on the development of diabetic retinopathy. A Scottish study gave results showing that alcohol has a severe adverse effect on diabetic retinopathy, particularly in the advancement of macular oedema and the development of proliferative retinopathy. Two other studies, however, one from the Veneto region in Italy and the other from Wisconsin, have shown that alcohol intake is not associated with deterioration of retinopathy, and indeed in the younger patients may well have a protective effect. These controversial results may be explained by the different drinking habits and the preferred type of alcoholic drinks in these countries.

c *Smoking cigarettes* The effect of smoking cigarettes is even more difficult to assess. The devastating effect of smoking on macrovascular disease is well recognised but its impact on microvascular disease is not so well documented and evidence has not always been consistent. Smoking increases the risk of albuminuria and thus almost certainly causes microvascular changes in the retina as well, whereas other studies have shown recently that smoking cigarettes has no adverse effect on the retina except in younger people. By contrast, Dodson showed that progression from non-proliferative diabetic retinopathy to proliferative diabetic retinopathy was more likely in elderly women who smoked.

d *Contraceptive pill* The contraceptive pill has also been incriminated in causing advancement of retinopathy. We have seen several cases which have all occurred with the high dose progesterone pill. In a case with mild retinopathy, stopping the pill resulted, within several months, in improvement of retinopathy and reduction in the leakage seen on the fluorescein angiogram (fig 1.2). It is unclear whether the modern low level hormone pill has enough thrombogenic activity to cause such advancement of retinopathy. The effect of hormone replacement therapy is as yet uncertain.

c Aspirin Drugs such as aspirin or calcium dobesilate (Doxium) are known to decrease thrombogenic activity but whether this is of any benefit in the prevention of diabetic retinopathy is still under discussion. The Early Treatment Diabetic Retinopathy Study (ETDRS) group investigated the effect of aspirin intake on the formation or advancement of existing diabetic retinopathy. The study concluded that there was no beneficial effect from aspirin.

2 Internal factors

Internal factors include age, arterial hypertension, lipids, nephropathy, pregnancy, and pituitary abnormalities.

Age Age dictates, to a large extent, the type of retinopathy. The younger group usually have type I diabetes and develop proliferative retinopathy whereas the older group have type II diabetes and develop macular oedema. The rate of progression differs. In the younger group advancement of proliferative diabetic retinopathy can be rapid and it was this group that was amenable to pituitary ablation in the years before panretinal photocoagulation was established.

b Hypertension and lipids Arterial hypertension is well known to cause deterioration of diabetic retinopathy. Hypercholesterolaemia is also a risk factor in type II diabetes mellitus along with arterial hypertension (fig 1.3). High blood pressure itself is often related to diabetic kidney disease, and it may be the hypertension that results in formation of macular oedema in the presence of diabetic kidney problems. Thus, in recent years the angiotensin converting enzyme

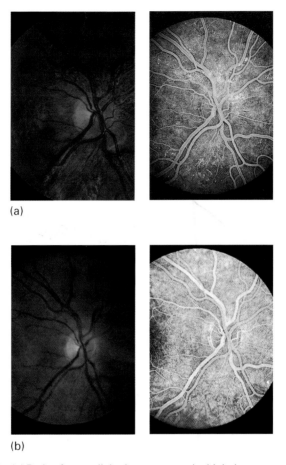

Figure 1.2   (a) Retina from a diabetic woman on the high dose contraceptive pill, and accompanying fluorescein angiogram; (b) one year after stopping taking the pill the situation has improved

inhibitor was found to be the antihypertensive agent of choice in such cases.

○ *Diabetic nephropathy*   Diabetic nephropathy aggravates diabetic retinopathy, especially macular oedema, and this may be mediated through the increase in blood pressure, fibrinogen levels, and raised lipoproteins. The early and adequate control of arterial hypertension has a favourable

8

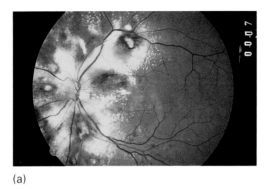

(a)

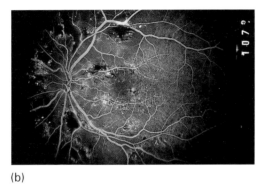

(b)

Figuro 1.3 (a) Retina showing combined retinopathy and severe hypertension; (b) fluorescein angiogram. Note the hard exudates even on the nasal
side of the optic disc. There are almost no microaneurysms temporal to the
fovea. This indicates a major influence from arterial hypertension

effect on the progression of diabetic retinopathy and macular
oedema. The effect of various methods of control of renal
failure on the course of visual acuity is illustrated in table
1.3.

The visual outcome is best with renal transplantation with
or without a combined pancreatic graft. Deterioration of
visual acuity most often occurs associated with haemodialysis.
The beneficial effect of renal transplantation may be
explained by the better control of arterial hypertension and
its influence on the formation of macular oedema. Fig 1.4

Table 1.3 The course of visual acuity associated with different modes of treatment for renal failure in diabetic patients

	Percentage of patients	
	Improved or stable	Worse
Haemodialysis ($n=29$)	38	62
Peritoneal dialysis ($n=18$)	83	17
Renal graft ($n=45$)	89	11
Renal + pancreatic graft ($n=34$)	88	12

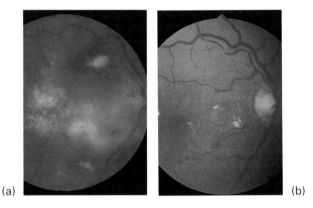

(a)   (b)

Figure 1.4 Retina of patient in renal failure: (a) before renal failure and (b) 12 months after the onset of renal failure. Note the increase in macular oedema

illustrates the aggravation of diabetic maculopathy within one year of the onset of renal failure which was treated with haemodialyses. Focal or grid photocoagulation in those severe cases can barely do more than control the situation; until a renal graft has succeeded the retina will not dry out or the response to photocoagulation improve.

d Pregnancy Pregnancy may accelerate the formation and advancement of diabetic retinopathy which may need photocoagulation at frequent intervals to control the progress. Important factors for the acceleration of the natural history of diabetic retinopathy during pregnancy are pregnancy per se, arterial hypertension, hyperglycaemia, rapid normalisation of blood glucose levels, duration of diabetes mellitus, and stage of diabetic retinopathy at baseline. Therefore, for diabetic women it is recommended to plan pregnancy in advance, and if necessay to normalise blood glucose levels slowly over a period of 6–8 months before conception. Photocoagulation should be performed during pregnancy according to the usual guidelines in spite of the possibility of spontaneous regression of macular oedema post partum. If the patient is already pregnant, normalisation of blood glucose is important and intensive surveillance of diabetic retinopathy every two months is needed.

Pituitary abnormalities It was an early observation that in diabetic individuals who have pituitary abnormalities such as low levels of growth hormone, for example, in pituitary dwarfs, and following pituitary gland infarction or ablation, proliferative diabetic retinopathy is rare. Today we know that many of the effects of growth hormone are mediated by insulin like growth factor (IGF). IGF has been found in elevated levels in the vitreous gel of patients with proliferating diabetic retinopathy. Another study by our own group revealed IGF receptors in diabetic epiretinal membranes. There seems therefore to be evidence for endocrinological effects on the formation of proliferative diabetic retinopathy. It is assumed that IGF is a part of the angiogenic factor that was postulated by Michaelson and Ashton in the 1950s. By contrast, in acromegaly, where growth hormone levels are high, diabetic retinopathy also tends to be mild; this may be explained by the fact that severe hyperglycaemia is uncommon in acromegaly. Pituitary ablation was the only method of controlling high risk proliferative diabetic retinopathy before the advent of panretinal photocoagulation (fig 1.5).

11

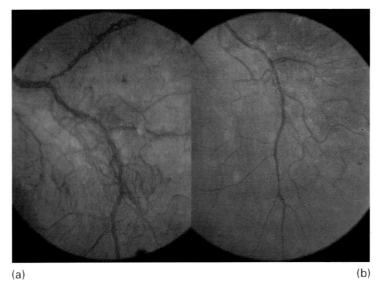

(a)   (b)

Figure 1.5 (a) Retina before pituitary ablation; (b) six months after completion of pituitary ablation there is regression of NVE

Ocular factors

The ocular factors that modify the natural history of diabetic retinopathy include high myopia, glaucoma, choroidal atrophy, posterior vitreous detachment, cataract surgery, and rubeosis iridis.

High myopia, glaucoma, choroidal atrophy Extensive myopia with choroidal degeneration, advanced glaucoma, and extensive old chorioretinopathy all protect against proliferative diabetic retinopathy; they probably act in the same way as panretinal photocoagulation by reducing the metabolic needs of the retina. In patients with choroidal atrophy in one eye proliferative retinopathy may only be observed in the fellow eye. On top of an atrophic glaucomatous disc new vessels rarely develop.

Posterior vitreous detachment Spontaneous posterior vitreous detachment and posterior vitreous detachment resulting from vitrectomy may prevent the progression of proliferative diabetic retinopathy because of the missing scaffold for forward new vessels, although not uncommonly small abortive neovascular outgrowths of new vessels which resemble raspberries may develop; these may cause recurrent vitreous haemorrhage. In addition, new vessels may creep along the retinal surface as flat new vessels. If neovascularisation reaches forward from the retina and spreads on the posterior face of the detached vitreous gel, haemorrhage into the gap between the hyaloid and the retina may occur. This haemorrhage precludes retinal photocoagulation and usually takes a long time to reabsorb. Thus, this form has a poor prognosis and requires early vitrectomy.

Cataract surgery The formation of cataracts may obscure developing treatable diabetic retinopathy and thus seriously alter the prognosis. Removal of a cataract even with a small incision technique and phacoemulsification may aggravate both existing macular oedema and proliferative diabetic retinopathy, and may hasten the onset of rubeosis iridis. Even anterior hyaloidal fibrovascular proliferation, which is common in vitrectomised phakic diabetic eyes, has been observed after uncomplicated cataract surgery in diabetic eyes (fig 1.6). Therefore, if the cataract is not too dense retinopathy should be treated properly before cataract surgery. The intention to perform early photocoagulation after cataract surgery is often prevented by a poor view in eyes with postoperative fibrinous uveitis. In diabetic individuals it is too easy to end up in a situation where anterior fibrinous deposits and an opaque capsule obscure the view and prevent adequate laser treatment. The best results of cataract surgery in diabetic patients are, however, in those with no diabetic retinopathy, with treated quiescent non-proliferative diabetic retinopathy, or with adequately treated macular oedema.

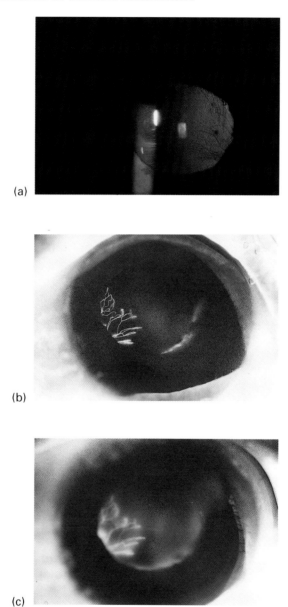

(a)

(b)

(c)

Figure 1.6 (a) Anterior segment showing a vessel lying on the posterior surface of the capsule in a pseudophakic eye; (b) fluorescein angiogram. This vessel is derived from the peripheral retina. (c) Late phase angiogram reveals leakage from the anterior hyaloidal fibrovascular proliferation

Iris neovascularisation Once iris neovascularisation has developed there is a high risk of losing the eye from secondary glaucoma and finally phthisis bulbi. Rubeosis iridis is a sign of rapid progression of proliferative diabetic eye disease. Therefore, once rubeosis iridis has been detected, full scatter panretinal photocoagulation is needed urgently to prevent the eye from becoming blind and painful.

2 Lasers

The power of light and of the sun has been appreciated since time immemorial. In ancient Greece, Apollo was the god of light (fig 2.1), and the sun was personified by a special deity called Helios. A flash of light from Helios's eyes was said to be so bright that it could pierce his golden helmet. The ophthalmic consequences of excessive light were first described in Plato's *Phaidon*, where Socrates compares the danger to the soul which could be blinded by the search for knowledge with that to the eyes which could be blinded by looking at an eclipse of the sun.

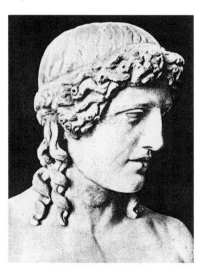

Figure 2.1 Apollo, the god of light. (Reproduced with permission of the Louvre)

Bonetus of Geneva in 1640 was the first to warn of eclipse blindness. The damaging effect of light has therefore been recognised for a considerable length of time. The development of lasers provides us with a more powerful and concentrated light source. Their technical development was preceded by science fiction accounts such as HG Wells's book *The war of the worlds* published in 1897. He depicted weapons in space shining a light beam capable of destroying buildings and armoured vehicles. Later in 1952, in the science fiction cartoon *Dan Dare—pilot of the future* published in the comic magazine *The Eagle*, the hero used laser weapons to destroy and kill (fig 2.2).

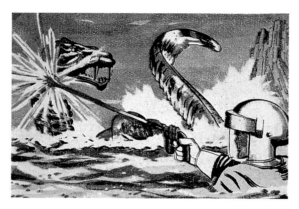

Figure 2.2 Dan Dare, one of the first laser users. (Reproduced with permission of Hulton Deutsch)

It was not, however, until 1960 that Maiman built the first working laser. This used a flash of light to stimulate a ruby crystal. Within three years this type of laser was being used in ophthalmology and since that time we have had a profusion of different sources and colours of laser light. These lasers have been accompanied by an equally impressive diversity of therapeutic applications and this trend is likely to continue in the future.

The recognition that light damage to the retina may have a beneficial therapeutic effect was first recognised by the German ophthalmologist Gerd Meyer-Schwickerath (fig 2.3). His publication in 1949 was the basis for the development of the field of retinal photocoagulation.

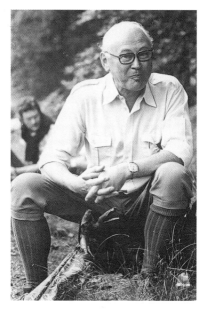

Figure 2.3 Professor G Meyer-Schwickerath introduced retinal photo-coagulation to ophthalmology. (Photograph courtesy of the family)

Description of lasers

The word "LASER" is an acronym for **L**ight **A**mplification by **S**timulated **E**mission of **R**adiation. Under certain circumstances, all matter can emit radiation but only a small proportion of radiation is within the visible part of the electromagnetic spectrum.

Radiation from any source is emitted when an electron returns from a high energy level to a lower energy level. The radiation is released in discrete energy packets called photons. When the wavelength of radiation is between 380 and 780 nm the emitted energy is visible as light (fig 2.4).

Most sources of visible light radiate energy at different wavelengths and at random time intervals. If the light source can be made to emit light of just one definite wavelength, which we call monochromatic light, one of the characteristics of a laser is met.

Figure 2.4   Light emitted from a lightbulb is emitted in all directions and is
incoherent

Box A   Characteristics of a laser
1 Monochromatic light 2 Spatial coherence 3 High density of electrons

Another characteristic of laser light is for all the high energy
electrons to return to the lower energy level at the same time,
so all the radiation is emitted in an instant. This requirement
is called the concept of spatial coherence and is more easily
understood if one considers that light travels in a waveform.
If, over a wide area, the peaks and troughs of the waves
correspond, and there is no interference, the waves are said
to be in phase (fig 2.5).

Monochromatic light can be achieved by the use of filters
or other optical devices, but most lasers use an optical
chamber, which is solid state or gas filled, to deliver
monochromatic light (fig 2.6). The chamber is of a specified
length, which is a multiple of the required wavelength, and
a standing wave is generated within a resonating cavity. Light
is bounced backwards and forwards from mirrors at each
end. When the laser is fired a certain amount is allowed to
escape through an aperture which is a semi-reflective mirror
at one end (fig 2.5).

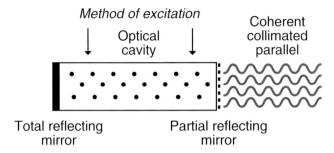

Figure 2.5 The optical cavity: the method of excitation is on the side of the cavity with the coherent collimated parallel rays emitted through the partial reflecting mirror

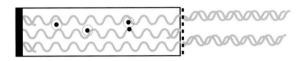

Figure 2.6 A gas tube laser with a mirror at each end. The right hand mirror is semi-reflective and allows the coherent collimated parallel rays to pass through it. The light within the optical cavity is reflected backwards and forwards, picking up photons from the excited gas molecules

The main problem in making a laser is not producing monochromatic light but ensuring that the light is emitted at the same phase. We have already determined that light is radiated during the return of an electron to a lower energy level, so the first requirement is to get at least 50% of the electrons in a high energy state; this is called inversion. Unfortunately most materials, although readily absorbing energy, allow the electrons to return to their resting state almost immediately, whereas the high energy state has to be maintained for effectiveness of laser light.

In addition to a gas filled tube, a ruby crystal slightly contaminated with chromium will provide a sufficiently long half life for electrons in an excited state to produce a laser. Energy can be transferred to a ruby crystal by a light source, a process called optical pumping, to produce a high preponderance of electrons in an activated state (fig 2.7).

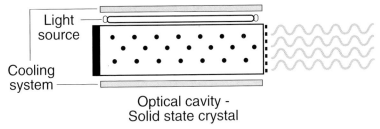

Figure 2.7   The exciting agent is the light source; this lies to the side of the optical cavity, and in this diagram the optical cavity is a solid state crystal. Surrounding the optical cavity is a cooling system

When most electrons are in higher energy levels the electron population is said to be inverted—called population inversion. The ruby crystal absorbs energy readily from a light source but it is the chromium contaminant that emits the laser light. Energy is transferred from the ruby to the chromium which has a high energy level and a long half life, and is said to be metastable.

All commercially produced lasers contain substances that have the property of sustaining an inverted population of electrons. The electrons are excited to a high energy state either by optically pumping the system or by electrical means (fig 2.8) If the laser releases all the energy from the inverted population each time the laser fires the laser is said to be pulsed, such as with a neodymium:yttrium–aluminium–garnet (Nd:YAG) laser. Conversely if only part of the energy

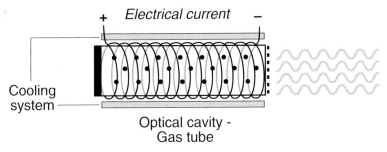

Figure 2.8   An optical cavity containing gas: this has an electrical current surrounding the optical cavity; surrounding this is a cooling system

is released, and then as quickly as it is released the source is reactivated, the laser is described as a continuous wave laser. The Nd:YAG laser is most useful when very high energies are required as in photodisruption procedures. Such high energy emissions can only be sustained for microseconds. A continuous wave laser is a laser that is used at lower energy levels and provides energy for photocoagulation.

Lasers in ophthalmology

In practical terms the lasers used in clinical ophthalmological practice can be subdivided into those for photocoagulation and those for disruption. In those for photocoagulation a chromophore absorbs the light converting the laser energy into heat. If the temperature rise reaches a certain critical level coagulation of the tissue will occur. A chromophore is not required for photodisruptor laser systems; instead an ultrashort pulse of light is targeted at the tissue, and at suprathreshold energy densities plasma formation will occur. In this way the tissue is disrupted mechanically.

Photocoagulators

The continuous wave lasers include argon blue–green, argon green, krypton red, adjustable dye, and the modern diode lasers. The introduction of the dye laser has allowed a range of visible wavelengths to be selected. Most continuous wave lasers, except the diode type, make use of a laser tube, which is a resonating chamber containing emitting argon or krypton gas. This tube is activated to laser activity by a surrounding electrical current. The photons released are rebounded between two mirrors at the very end of the tube. With passage through the tube photons are released until sufficient power is obtained to penetrate the partially silvered mirror at one end of the resonating chamber. The continuous beam thus produced is filtered to allow only a small amount through, and in most systems this acts as the aiming beam of the laser. More modern laser systems use a separate diode laser beam for aiming which is regarded as safer for the laser user. The described filter is mechanically removed at the time of laser firing, allowing the full beam to pass. The laser is traditionally attached to a modified slitlamp microscope via a fibreoptic arm and directed into the eye. The direction can be altered with a micromanipulator and the spot size of the laser beam adjusted by convex lenses to alter the convergence angle of the beam. The convergence angle of this type of laser varies between 4 and 5°. The smallest spot size with these lasers is in the region of 50 μm with a range up to 2000 μm.

Recently laser indirect ophthalmoscope delivery systems were developed which are considered very useful for the treatment of the peripheral retina, that is, peripheral retinal breaks or retinopathy of prematurity.

Examples of laser systems that use solid state electronics as an energy source are the semiconductor diode laser (fig 2.9) and the doubled frequency Nd:YAG laser (532 nm). The semiconductor diode laser uses one or several diodes to emit the radiation at 810 nm and is electrically pumped (figs 2.9, 2.10 and 2.11). The advantages of the diode lasers are significant and may make the more expensive, much larger, water cooled, argon laser obsolete in the future. The diode laser is portable with the approximate size of a video recorder, and can be simply attached to a standard slitlamp microscope. There is no necessity for a three phase electricity supply and the diode laser can be powered with either batteries or 13 amp mains supply. The infrared diode laser is the only continuous wave system that radiates outside the visible spectrum; this means that a mechanical shutter flap is not required during treatment. Instead a permanent barrier filter is placed between the operator and the laser mechanism, so filtering out any reflected infrared light. The use of this barrier filter allows continuous visualisation of the retina as the burn develops, facilitating a more accurate assessment of the end point of the laser burn. This is in contrast to the argon laser which precludes visualisation of the developing burn by the mechanical shutter flap. The convergence angle is much greater than with the gas filled tube lasers and can be as much as 23°. The smallest spot size is 75 µm with a

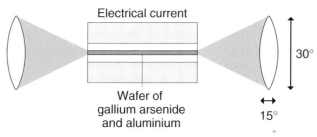

Figure 2.9 Diode laser showing the aluminium–gallium arsenide crystal electrically driven; there is also a conical emitted laser light at the 810 nm frequency

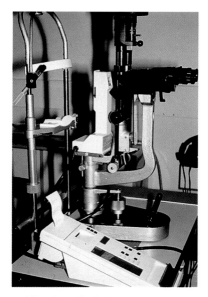

Figure 2.10   A Keeler Microlase diode laser

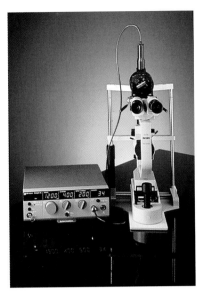

Figure 2.11   An Oculight diode laser. (Photograph provided by IRIS Medical)

range up to 1000 μm. The aiming beam is provided by a coaxial red diode laser.

Laser diodes are special types of semiconductor junctions. Semiconductors are crystalline materials in which, at ambient temperatures, electrical resistance is midway between that of an insulator (for example, plastic) and a conductor (for example, a metal). In all materials electrons can exist at a number of energy levels. Electrons at a lower energy level occupy a region called the valence band. There is also a smaller population of electrons that occupy a higher energy band, which is termed the conduction band. Electrons in this band are delocalised and are not associated with a single nucleus. The relative distribution of electrons in these bands confers the properties of a conductor or an insulator. The difference in energies of the two bands, termed the "band gap," is small in a semiconductor. It therefore requires a small input of energy to enable electrons to move to the higher level and for conduction to occur.

The electronic properties of semiconductors can be modified by "doping." Doping refers to the introduction of "foreign" atoms into the crystal lattice during its synthesis. Since the first laser diode was introduced, there have been many advances in device efficiency. The use of heterojunctions has resulted in increased output power, with lower laser threshold current. A heterojunction is a semiconductor junction between two different materials. One heterojunction used in diode lasers is that between gallium arsenide (GaAs) and gallium aluminium arsenide (GaAlAs). This is the laser that is currently used in ophthalmology. It can be prepared to emit anywhere in the region 750–950 nm, although the emission of high power diodes (1 watt) is at present restricted to the near infrared region (780–840 nm).

The active layer of a gallium aluminium arsenide laser diode is 0·2 μm thick and composed of GaAs; it is sandwiched between two layers of GaAlAs 1 μm thick. The dimensions of a laser diode are typically $0·5 \times 0·2 \times 0·1$ mm.

As a consequence of the introduction of diode lasers in ophthalmology, argon laser technology has improved greatly in recent years. The most recent argon laser systems are now designed to be portable and can be attached to standard mains. The time interval for renewal of the laser tube was lengthened, cutting down on the cost for running such a system. The most compact argon lasers are now the size of a Samsonite case but are still quite heavy, weighing in the region of 30 kg.

Photodisruptors

This class of lasers was introduced to ophthalmology simultaneously by Aron Rosa and Franz Fankhauser in 1977. These lasers produce very high energy pulses that are sufficient to disrupt intraocular tissues and membranes. The predominant photodisruptor with widespread use in clinical ophthalmology is the Nd:YAG laser (1064 nm) (fig 2.12).

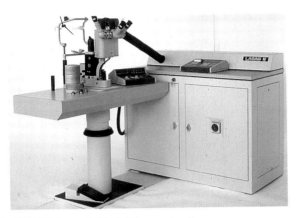

Figure 2.12 Nd:YAG laser: LASAG Microruptor II

This is an optically driven system, and contains a crystal of yttrium–aluminium–garnet with about 5% neodymium incorporated in the crystal. The Nd:YAG laser delivers energy at very high levels and results in plasma formation. A plasma means a strip of all electrons from a parent molecule and this effect is used therapeutically to disrupt intraocular tissues, that is, to punch holes.

Box B	**Lasers in ophthalmology**	
Type	*Method of pumping*	*Wavelength (nm)*
Ruby	Optically pulsed	694
Argon blue	Electrical continuous wave	488
Argon green	Electrical continuous wave	514
Krypton	Electrical continuous wave	647
Dye	Electrical continuous wave	Variable
Nd:YAG	Optically pulsed	1064
Nd:YAG	Doubled frequency pulsed	532
Excimer	Optically pulsed	193
Diode	Electrical continuous wave	810
Nd:YLF	Optically pulsed	1053

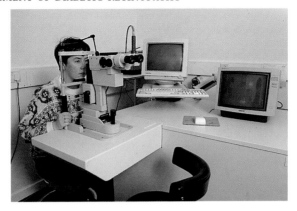

Figure 2.13 Computer driven Nd:YLF picosecond laser produced by ILS (Intelligent Laser Systems)

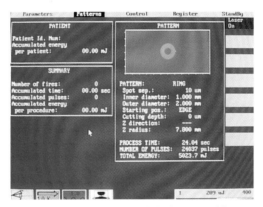

Figure 2.14 Computer screen of the Nd:YLF picosecond laser

More recently the so called picosecond laser, a neodymium:yttrium–lithium–fluoride (Nd:YLF) system has been introduced which is capable of producing 1000 micropulses per second at a wavelength of 1053 nm. With this laser technique continuous cutting of intraocular tissue with a variety of computer modulated patterns is possible (figs 2.13 and 2.14).

Xenon light photocoagulator

The xenon light photocoagulator (fig 2.15) was developed by the German ophthalmologist Gerd Meyer-Schwickerath in 1954 and was generally used before the argon laser became available. This first photocoagulator was a milestone of photocoagulation technique in its period and made photocoagulation independent of sunlight and weather conditions. Some ophthalmologists still use it currently to treat some resistant forms of proliferative diabetic retinopathy, but in general it is out of use. The latest xenon photocoagulator

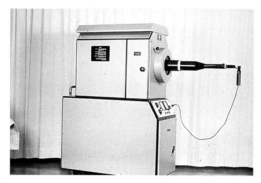

Figure 2.15   Early model of a xenon light photocoagulator as produced by Zeiss, West Germany

(fig 2.16) was air cooled and semiportable. It was mainly used for retinal photocoagulation in the prelaser era and in the 1970s. Finally, it even provided options for modification for endophotocoagulation. The viewing system consists of a modified direct ophthalmoscope with a mechanical shutter which is lowered when the xenon photocoagulator is fired. The energy source is white xenon light which produces a retinal burn similar to the standard continuous wave lasers used today. The minimum spot size is larger than that of most laser photocoagulators (fig 2.17), measured in degrees of arc rather than micrometres. The range of most types of xenon photocoagulators is variable from 3° to 8°. The exposure time and other power settings for the xenon photocoagulator are usually greater than those used for

29

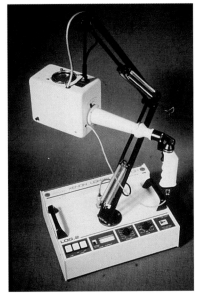

Figure 2.16   O'Malley xenon light photocoagulator from the 1970s

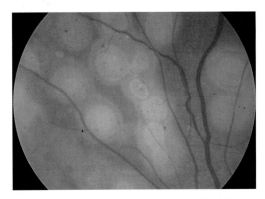

Figure 2.17 Typical photocoagulation burns with the xenon light photocoagulator

continuous wave lasers. As a consequence the retinal burn produced by the xenon photocoagulator is usually a full thickness burn of the sensory retina, and this, together with the larger spot size, causes more side effects than comparable treatment with standard lasers.

As a result of the size and intensity required to produce a retinal burn ocular anaesthesia is generally required. Most patients will require a retrobulbar anaesthetic and some patients may need a general anaesthetic.

Laser effects on the eye

All electromagnetic radiation can be reflected, transmitted, or absorbed. For the laser to be therapeutically effective within the eye it needs to be transmitted through the ocular media so that it can enter the eye and be absorbed by a chromophore.

The possible effect of lasers on the eye depends on the site of absorption and the temperature rise at this site. The effects are photochemical, photoirradiation (raises the temperature by only a few degrees centigrade), photocoagulation (raises the temperature by 30°C and more) (fig 2.18), and photodisruption (raises the temperature up to 20 000°C).

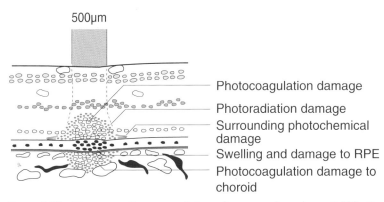

500µm

Photocoagulation damage

Photoradiation damage

Surrounding photochemical damage

Swelling and damage to RPE

Photocoagulation damage to choroid

Figure 2.18 Diagrammatic representation of an argon laser burn at 500 µm spot size. This shows the burn centred on the pigment epithelium and the diminishing effect of the heat dissipated on the surrounding structures

Photochemical effect

The effect of the light on a tissue varies according to the amount of energy absorbed. During daylight hours the retina is constantly being irradiated with visible light, yet this does not have the same effect as a laser because the energy and temporal aspects are different. In the noon day sun, the background luminance levels vary between 0.01 mW/cm^2 and 0.1 mW/cm^2 of retina. At these radiances a photochemical change occurs in the retina, converting *cis*-retinol to *trans*-retinol, so initiating the perception of light.

Although photochemical reactions can result in injury to the eye, for example, arc flash photokeratitis, most light damage contains a thermal component. Irradiation even at low levels, causing only small rises in temperature, can produce damage. Fortunately most of this is transient and recovery is the rule. Exposure to this level of irradiation has been documented as occurring during laser therapy to both the laser operator and the patient. In the patient, areas of retina adjacent to those being targeted absorb scattered light and this mechanism probably accounts for some of the transient visual loss experienced by the patient. Similarly triton defects have been documented in clinicians following laser treatment to their patients as a result of the reflected laser light from the aiming beam. With modern laser systems this is prevented by using an additional coaxial diode laser beam for targeting.

Photochemical damage will also occur in areas adjacent to a visible burn on the retina. The further from the burn, the greater the chance of this being reversible, but in the more adjacent areas this damage will be permanent. This is important to remember when treating in proximity to the foveola.

Photoirradiation

If the temperature rises by only a few degrees, there may be damage to the tissue without any apparent visible whitening in the retina. This will occur in the retina when low dose irradiation is applied, if the laser is defocused, or in the area surrounding a visible laser burn. Although there is no immediate visible damage, in time structural changes at the retinal pigment epithelium may be seen. This damage accounts for the increase in size of a laser burn which may be seen some months after the laser treatment. This enlargement of burn size as a result of photoirradiation is often greater in myopic patients who have a less pigmented retinal pigment epithelium (RPE).

Photocoagulation

Photocoagulation results in a visible burn in the retina, accompanied by a rise in temperature to about 30°C.

Most of the therapeutic effects of lasers are the result of photocoagulation. To photocoagulate the retina, energy needs to be absorbed in sufficient quantities to cause a significant local temperature rise. An average luminance from a continuous wave laser, set at 1 mW, during photocoagulation is 10 000 mW/cm^2. This is sufficient to raise the temperature to 30°C and to coagulate the RPE. Obviously the temporal relationship is important when considering the effects of radiation on the eye, but in general damage can occur in fractions of a second with high levels of irradiance, but may not develop for some hours at lower levels of irradiance.

Electromagnetic radiation can be reflected, transmitted, or absorbed. For the continuous wave lasers to be therapeutically effective, the target tissue must absorb that particular wavelength. Within the eye, the major absorbing tissues are melanin, haemoglobin, and xanthophyll pigment.

Photodisruption

If the temperature of the target is raised to in the region of 20 000°C for a short period of time (nanoseconds) and very accurately focused, then photodisruption occurs. The centre of this reaction produces a plasma that disrupts the molecules of the tissue and the tissue "evaporates." This process of disruption may be produced by neodymium laser systems which are currently available in two variants: the nanosecond Nd:YAG laser and the picosecond high frequency Nd:YLF laser which can produce 1000 pulses/second. These lasers are more commonly used in the anterior segment of the eye, but may also be used to divide or cut vitreous bands or sheets, or to open the posterior hyaloid face in cases of premacular subhyaloid haemorrhages.

Physical parameters of lasers

The laser console contains dials that allow the physical parameters governing energy delivery to be varied. If wavelength is excluded these parameters are spot size, duration of application, and power. The "power" is the rate at which the energy is delivered. The units of energy are recorded in joules (J); the power is joules per unit of time:

$$\text{Power} = \frac{\text{Energy}}{\text{Time}}$$

If energy is in joules, and time in seconds, power is measured in watts (W). So without altering the power setting, the energy delivered to the eye can be varied by duration of exposure.

For example,

Power = 300 mW
Time $(t) = 0\cdot1$ s
Energy delivered to the eye = 30 mJ.

If time is changed to $t = 0\cdot2$ s, energy delivered to the eye is 60 mJ. Similarly if the power and duration are kept constant, but the spot size is varied, the energy is varied reciprocally from the formula:

$$\text{Energy density} = \text{Power}.$$

Method of delivery

The most common delivery system consists of a slitlamp microscope attached to a laser generating system (see fig 2.11). The slitlamp microscope is a modified commercial unit with perhaps higher magnification, a micromanipulator, and, if needed, a mechanical shutter flap that drops when the laser is fired. In the semiconductor diode laser, however, the operator is protected from the laser light by optical filters and no mechanical shutter mechanism is required. In the latest generation of argon lasers there is a filter set in position when the laser is activated which protects the observer from reflected blue–green light. The aiming beam is provided by a separate red coaxial diode laser.

The console on the laser usually contains a safety on–off switch, spot size, power, and exposure time dials, and an exposure counter. The spot size with most systems is either continuously or discretely variable from 50 µm to 2000 µm. Similarly the power and duration of burn can be varied. Many lasers have a switch to activate a rapid fire repeat mode. This allows continuous rapid firing of the laser by constant activation of the foot pedal for panretinal photocoagulation. The exposure and interval time are both adjustable.

The laser is directed into the patient's eye through a lens system, most often contact, rarely non-contact. There is a wide range of contact lenses available varying from the classic Goldmann three mirror or fundus lens to a variety of panfundoscopic lenses, designed to treat particular areas of the eye. Hand held or supported non-contact lenses with a special coating such as the 60 dioptre (D), 78 D, or 90 D aspherical lenses are rarely used.

Lasers can also be applied through indirect ophthalmoscopes (fig 2.19). An indirect lens is used, which should have a special coating that matches the laser wavelength employed, and varying the power of this lens will slightly modify the spot size at the retina. The spot size can also be varied by moving the indirect ophthalmoscope either away from or towards the eye.

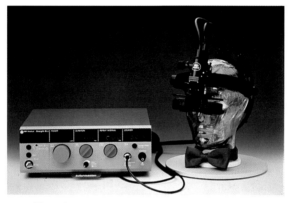

Figure 2.19 The laser indirect ophthalmoscope attached to the semiconductor diode laser Oculight SLX (IRIS Medical)

With the xenon photocoagulator or indirect laser ophthalmoscope, during treatment the eyelids are held open with a lid speculum and intermittent corneal irrigation is needed to prevent corneal desiccation and to provide good visualisation of the retina. There are, in addition, other methods of delivering laser to the eye. It can be applied through endoprobes to the retina during vitrectomy, by a probe trans-sclerally to the retina, and via a probe trans-sclerally to the ciliary body (with a specially designed cyclophotocoagulation probe, that is, the IRIS Medical G-Probe). The trans-scleral application forms are limited to those lasers with wavelength characteristics that allow for trans-scleral passage of the laser beam, such as the diode and the Nd:YAG laser.

Effect of different laser parameters

The settings on the laser should be chosen according to the intensity of burn required and altered to suit the patient and ocular characteristics. The effects of laser therapy are multifactorial and depend on the many parameters affecting laser–tissue interactions. Central to this interaction are transmission of laser energy through the ocular media, relative absorption characteristics of the eye, and the wavelength of the light. Other independent variables include power, duration, and size of burn, plus the total number of burns and the total area treated.

Melanin is responsible for absorbing most of the laser energy in the eye and is contained in the retinal pigment epithelium and in lesser quantities in the melanocytes of the choroid. Other pigments that need to be considered are xanthophyll in the ocular lens and fovea, and haemoglobin and other pigments found in the lens and retina of the ageing eye (see box C).

An understanding of the target cell when treating diabetic retinopathy with the laser is important to minimise the adverse effects of lasering. When the target is the retinal pigment epithelium, as is usually the case in diabetic retinopathy, the ideal reaction is one that just blanches the retinal pigment epithelium. This is called a threshold burn. This holds for focal, grid, and panretinal photocoagulation.

Box C   Absorbing pigments in the eye

1 Melanin in the retinal pigment epithelium
2 Xanthophyll in the fovea
3 Haemoglobin within red blood cells
4 Choroidal and scleral melanocytes
5 Lipofuscin in ageing eyes

Light burns will minimise the damage to the sensory retina, Bruch's membrane, and choroid, and reduce the risk of choroidal detachment following sessions of panretinal treatment with up to 1000 burns.

Argon laser

The argon blue–green laser system emits light over a narrow band width, but through six wavelengths. The main peaks are at 488 and 514 nm, respectively, in the blue and green part of the spectrum. In the modern argon laser systems, the blue wavelength can be excluded and this option is generally advocated because of the potential patient and operator photochemical damage, as a result of absorption in the xanthophyll pigment. The "blue," however, contributes about 40% of the energy output of the argon laser, so for rare occasions when high energy is required the combined wavelengths may be necessary.

Table 2.1 Absorption of different lasers in ocular pigments

Laser	Wavelength (nm)	RPE	Haemoglobin	Xanthophyll
Argon	488	+ + + +	+ +	+ +
Argon	514	+ + + +	+ +	+
Krypton	647	+ +	−	−
Dye	577	+ + +	+ +	−
Dye	630	+ +	−	−
Diode	810	+	−	−

RPE = retinal pigment epithelium.

Retinal pigment epithelium

The argon laser is predominantly absorbed by the retinal pigment epithelium with a lesser absorption (about 40%) by the choroidal melanocytes (fig 2.20). Following delivery of a therapeutic burn the RPE immediately whitens. This can vary from a minimally whitish–grey burn to a progressively marble white burn. With very high intensity burns there is often a heaping up of the RPE at the margin of the burn, giving rise to a dark halo around the white burn. Even heavier burns may result in rupture of Bruch's membrane and choroidal vessels, and the subsequent haemorrhage may extend into the vitreous gel (fig 2.21).

Heat absorbed by the RPE is dissipated around the burn with transfer to the sensory retina, adjacent RPE, and choroid. This leads to a variable degree of destruction in these structures which is predominantly determined by intensity and dissipation of the burn. The lateral spread of heat to adjacent RPE cells decreases exponentially with distance but a mild, greyish threshold burn does not extend far (fig 2.22). There may, however, be sufficient uptake of heat to produce a delayed reaction in the RPE and this may be reflected clinically as enlargement of the area of RPE atrophy with time.

Haemoglobin

Argon laser in the blue or blue–green spectrum is absorbed by both oxyhaemoglobin and the reduced haemoglobin (deoxyhaemoglobin). Although the uptake of blue green energy is not as great as it is for melanin, it is still sufficient to allow for direct coagulation of leaking retinal micro-aneurysms or forward new vessels, but this needs a fair amount of energy (fig 2.23). More recent studies have shown that blanching the RPE underneath a retinal microaneurysm may be sufficient to treat leaking microaneurysms in the macular area. The difference in absorption of laser energies between oxyhaemoglobin and deoxyhaemoglobin is not clinically relevant.

Xanthophyll

The xanthophyll pigment lies in the inner and outer plexiform layers at the fovea and absorbs light of short

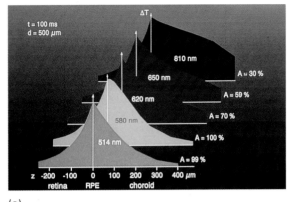

(a)

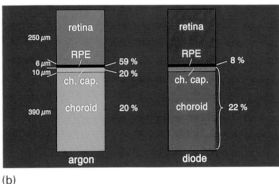

(b)

Figure 2.20 (a) Heat transmitted from the RPE following burns of different wavelengths. The transfer of heat occurs into both the retina and the choroid for the different wavelengths, ranging from 514 nm in the green argon band to 810 nm in the diode laser band. (b) The percentage absorption of light in the RPE, choriocapillary, and choroid between the argon laser and the diode laser. (Courtesy of Professor V Peter Gabel)

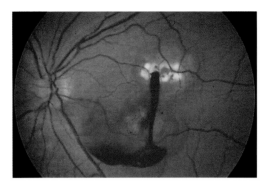

Figure 2.21   A heavy argon laser burn ruptured Bruch's membrane resulting in a vitreous haemorrhage

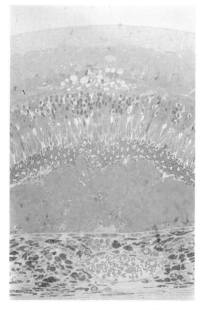

Figure 2.22   Histological preparation showing mild, greyish, threshold burn on the RPE

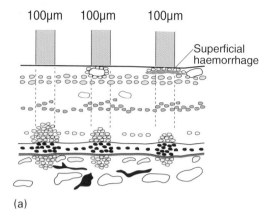

(a)

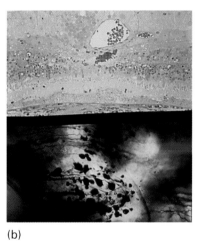

(b)

Figure 2.23   (a) Diagrammatic representation of the retina with, on the left, an argon laser burn of 100 μm spot size damaging the RPE with transmitted heat into the retina and choroid. The middle area shows the argon laser burn directed at a retinal blood vessel showing re-uptake in the surrounding tissue and reduced absorption at the level of the pigment epithelium. On the right a 100 μm burn aimed at a superficial haemorrhage again shows uptake in the nerve fibre layer and reduced reaction at the level of the RPE. (b) Top: an argon laser burn directed at a retinal blood vessel. Haemoglobin has absorbed the argon laser, and there is surrounding retinal damage. Bottom: on the flat mount preparation, the nerve fibre layers have been disrupted, and there is an accumulation of axoplasm at the end of the broken nerve fibre layer

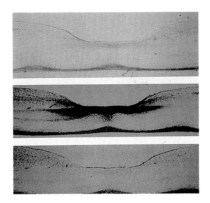

Figure 2.24 Histological preparation of the macular area, showing xanthophyll pigment in white light on the top, blue light in the middle, and green light below. This shows that the xanthophyll pigment absorbs blue light

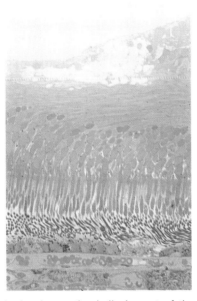

Figure 2.25 Uptake by the xanthophyll pigment of the argon laser, with destruction of the nerve fibre layer

wavelengths (fig 2.24). Absorption of the blue light component from the argon blue–green laser may cause a burn in the sensory retina during photocoagulation of the fovea, with significant visual loss (fig 2.25). Transfer of heat from the RPE to the sensory retina may cause changes in the internal limiting membrane with shrinkage and puckering of the macula. A further disadvantage with uptake in the sensory retina is the subsequent masking of the RPE by oedematous retina making it difficult to get sufficient uptake at the RPE. Occasionally uptake by the xanthophyll is exploited therapeutically in the direct treatment of retinal microaneurysms in the macular area responsible for macular oedema. This technique should, however, be limited to very rare indications because the horizontal damage within the sensory retina may outweigh the benefits of this treatment technique by far.

Krypton laser

The krypton laser emits light at two main peaks: 568·2 nm in the yellow and 647 nm in the red band. The red band contains most of the energy and is largely responsible for the photocoagulation effect. The krypton laser has certain advantages over the shorter wavelength lasers: there is less scattering of the laser light through the cornea and lens; vitreous opacities and blood are less of an obstacle with this laser; and there is much less "flash" to the patient during the procedure. The light from the krypton laser is absorbed predominantly by the melanin pigment in the RPE and choroid. Penetration is deeper with this laser than with the blue–green laser, and for this reason it is more painful to the patient when treatment is applied to the region peripheral to the vascular arcades. A major disadvantage with this laser is the small therapeutic window between a subthreshold and suprathreshold burn. At the same power setting, small regional variations in pigmentation of the RPE or choroid can significantly alter the appearance of a burn from a mild greyish burn to an intense marble white burn, perhaps with a choroidal haemorrhage. Similarly, the energy density may be adversely affected by defocusing the laser or tilting the contact lens.

Retinal pigment epithelium

Melanin in the RPE layer absorbs about 20% of the incident krypton laser energy and is considered to be responsible for the therapeutic effect in krypton laser photocoagulation. About 80% of the laser energy is, however, transmitted through the RPE and is absorbed by melanocytes in the choroid (see fig 2.20).

Thus, the appearance of the krypton burn is somewhat different to the argon burn, and with gentle applications of equivalent power it produces a much greyer type of reaction on the RPE. By increasing the power setting the greyness of the burn may not be enhanced to the marble white of the argon blue–green laser, and the end point is therefore more difficult to judge. This results from the more pronounced absorption by choroidal melanocytes. In the treatment of diabetic retinopathy, however, greyish threshold burns are most desirable.

Haemoglobin

The red krypton laser wavelength is not absorbed by haemoglobin and therefore, for focal macular laser treatment, this laser can only be used to coagulate RPE that is located directly underneath the leaking retinal vasculature (fig 2.26). Direct photocoagulation of retinal microaneurysms should not be attempted with this type of laser because no direct coagulation will occur within the lesion. Closure of the vascular lesion may only occur either by heat transfer from the underlying RPE or indirectly by inhibitory growth factors released by the stimulated RPE.

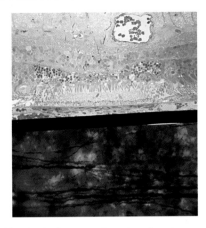

Figure 2.26 Top: histological preparation showing damage to the pigment epithelium by a krypton burn with no damage to the blood vessel and the surrounding area. Bottom: the intact nerve fibre layer, running across the vessel, confirming that there is no inner retinal damage with a krypton laser burn

Xanthophyll

Xanthophyll pigment only minimally absorbs krypton laser, and this effect can be clinically ignored (figs 2.27 and 2.28). This fact makes the krypton laser theoretically an ideal laser for treatment of lesions closely located to the fovea.

Dye laser

The adjustable wavelength dye laser allows for a wide range of laser wavelengths. The major wave bands that are used are the green at 514 nm, yellow at 577 nm, orange at 590 nm, and red at 630 nm. The treatment characteristics of the green together with the red are the same as those of the single wavelength argon and krypton laser systems. The advantages of the other wavelengths with the dye laser have not been proved clearly.

The orange wavelength has similar properties to that of the krypton red. This wavelength is minimally absorbed by

100μm Argon   100μm Krypton

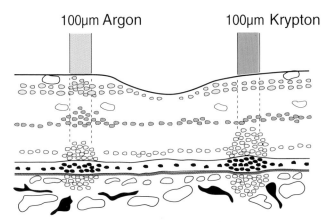

Figure 2.27 Diagrammatic representation of a 100 μm argon burn showing uptake in the xanthophyll pigment with the potential of destroying the nerve fibre layer and denervating the fovea. The corresponding krypton burn on the right shows the uptake in the pigment epithelium with transmission of krypton laser light through the xanthophyll pigment

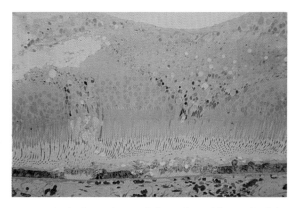

Figure 2.28 Histological specimen of the retina with, on the left, an argon laser burn showing inner retinal damage and, on the right, a krypton laser burn showing that it penetrates the xanthophyll pigment, producing a burn on the pigment epithelium

xanthophyll and haemoglobin. Conversely yellow is absorbed by haemoglobin but not xanthophyll; this may be ideal for direct coagulation of retinal microaneurysms located close to the fovea. On the other hand, as mentioned above, direct coagulation of these lesions does not appear to be necessary. Both yellow and orange wavelengths have similar intraocular transmission profiles.

Retinal pigment epithelium

Both yellow and orange wavelengths are preferentially absorbed by the RPE and produce equivalent burns at similar energy densities (see fig 2.20).

Haemoglobin

We have found that 577 nm has advantages in the treatment of haemoglobin containing structures that require lower energies to achieve "closure" of retinal microaneurysms and leaking capillaries. Direct closure of forward new vessels is also possible with this wavelength. When treating retinal microaneurysms close to the fovea, 577 nm has the added advantage of being minimally absorbed by xanthophyll, so preventing the possibility of injury to the adjacent Henle fibres.

Xanthophyll

Neither orange nor yellow wavelengths are significantly absorbed by xanthophyll.

Semiconductor diode laser

This laser has a wavelength of 810 nm and lies outside the visible spectrum in the near infrared region. As the laser beam is invisible, the patient is not aware of any flash of light during activation of the laser and this is an advantage in those patients who are photophobic with conventional lasers. The diode laser has similar absorption profiles to the krypton red laser and the therapeutic window is equally small. Differences in the density of choroidal melanocytes may lead to a variation of the laser burn. Even subthreshold burns have, however, shown efficacy in the treatment of proliferative diabetic retinopathy.

Retinal pigment epithelium

Most of the laser energy from the diode laser is absorbed by the pigment in the melanocytes of the choroid and only around 8% is absorbed by the RPE. This reduced absorption within the RPE may have advantages in decreasing secondary photoreceptor damage and faster restoration of the outer blood–ocular barrier (see fig 2.20).

Clinically the burn produced by the diode laser is similar to that produced by the krypton red laser and as with increasing energies the burn changes from grey to white–grey (fig 2.29).

Diode laser
500μm

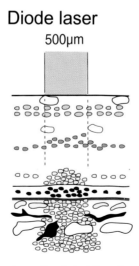

Figure 2.29 Diode laser burn directed at the pigment epithelium, showing the greater transmission of light with absorption by the melanocytes of the choroid

Haemoglobin

Haemoglobin does not absorb 810 nm light and, if the diode laser is to be used to treat retinal microaneurysms, either heat must be transferred from the RPE or release of inhibitory growth factors from the RPE must be induced. Alternatively energy uptake by the retinal microaneurysms or forward new vessels may be enhanced by preoperative intravenous injection of indocyanin green, which provides an ideal absorption peak at 795 nm.

Xanthophyll

Xanthophyll does not absorb 810 nm light significantly. Thus, the diode laser is also considered a theoretically ideal laser for foveal or parafoveal treatments.

Laser variables

There are a number of independent variables available on most laser machines. These include spot size, duration of exposure, and power.

Spot size

Most continuous wave lasers have a facility to vary the spot size from 50 μm to 2000 μm. This is achieved by simply varying the divergence of the emerging beam relative to the distance to the end point, taken at the level of the slitlamp microscope. It follows that the spot size can be further varied by defocusing the slitlamp microscope, or even using another type of contact lens. It is important to appreciate that defocusing the slitlamp microscope during lasering can cause a significant change in power density delivered to the retina

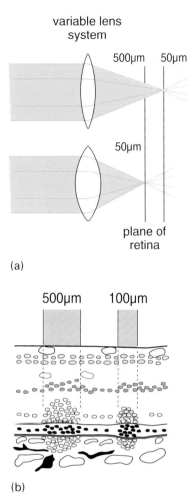

(a)

(b)

Figure 2.30 (a) The effect of changing the lens system on the converging beam emitted from a laser system, so that the position of the focal point of the laser is adjusted to the retina. (b) Diagrammatic representation of the change in the burn, defocusing from 100 to 500 μm

(fig 2.30). With the "Volk Area Centralis" lens and the Goldmann three mirror lens, the spot size at the retina is almost identical as dialled on the slitlamp microscope or the laser console, but for instance with the Rodenstock panfundoscope the retinal burn is 1·43 times enlarged; thus a dialled 200 μm burn appears as a 286 μm size burn on the retina. With the Volk Quadraspheric contact lens the spot size is double on the retina. With most lasers, defocusing the laser anteriorly causes the spot to enlarge. Conversely, defocusing the beam posteriorly minimises the burn and if the power is not adjusted will lead to a heavier burn (fig 2.31).

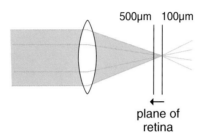

500μm 100μm

plane of
retina

Figure 2.31   The effect of defocusing the laser system so that if the 100 μm spot is focused on the plane of the retina, pushing the laser towards the patient, it will result in a larger spot size. Defocusing away from the patient will reduce the size of the spot, to its minimum—50 μm

If the ideal burn is taken as one that just blanches the RPE, then the effect of altering the size will be to change the power density and subsequent spread of heat generated. For a small burn with minimal blanching of the RPE, the spread of heat into the adjacent retina and choroid is minimal. The larger the burns the greater the spread (fig 2.32). In practical terms this means, when treating large areas of retina, that the burn size is made as large as possible with the proviso that the burn should not be unacceptably painful for the patient and not spread signficantly into the sensory retina. A 500 μm spot size on the retina is considered optimal for panretinal photocoagulation.

Power

The power output of ophthalmic lasers is measured in milliwatts (mW). The actual delivery of power depends on the transfer function and the power measured on the console

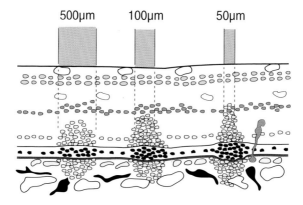

Figure 2.32   Diagrammatic representation of a 500, 100, and 50 μm spot size showing the increased energy uptake by the RPE. With a 50 μm spot size the high energy has caused disruption of choroidal blood vessels with bleeding into the retina

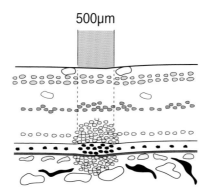

Figure 2.33   A gentle burn causing uptake by the pigment epithelium spreading into the retina and choroid. The retinal damage is mild and insufficient to cause disruption of horizontal connections in the retina, the nerve fibre layer, and the ganglion cell layer

is not necessarily what reaches the retina. In general the power setting should be as low as possible, being sufficient to cause only the desired reaction on the RPE or any other target tissue (fig 2.33). The severity of the burn should be closely monitored throughout the treatment session and the power altered as required. At low levels of energy, damage may not be clinically visible and the transfer of energy is at a photochemical level. If damage is done to the RPE cells it may be apparent only with fluorescein angiography as a small hyperfluorescent area, signifying disruption of the outer blood–retina barrier. Suprathreshold burns may not only cause disruption of Bruch's membrane and choroidal haemorrhages, but also coagulation of the layers of the sensory retina (fig 2.34). These complications can significantly reduce visual function (fig 2.35).

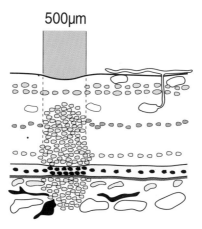

500μm

Figure 2.34   Diagrammatic representation of a moderate burn, showing that there is damage spreading into the inner retinal layers with greater damage to the horizontal connections in the retina; the heat has almost reached the ganglion cell layer

Energy transfer to adjacent structures can also be affected by other parameters besides the absolute energy delivered to the eye. Long wavelengths penetrate more deeply through the retina, affecting proportionally more choroidal cells (see fig 2.29). Conversely, a retinal vessel overlying an area to be photocoagulated may absorb sufficient light to transfer enough energy to coagulate the sensory retina (see fig 2.23). Similarly haemorrhage or pigment in the retina, if lasered, can absorb energy and shift the site of coagulation. Retreating over freshly treated RPE will reflect energy back up

500µm

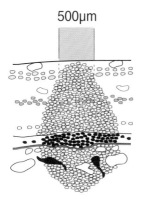

Figure 2.35 Diagrammatic representation of a heavier burn, showing the uptake of the nerve fibre layer and the ganglion cell layer; a corresponding loss of function will occur

into the sensory retina and in most cases this should be avoided.

If laser is applied at a later date over a previously treated area, the heat and damage profiles are altered as a result of the previous migration, following the initial burn, of pigment granules into the sensory retina and choroid (fig 2.36). Pigment may also disperse into the vitreous gel with the potential for converting into fibroblasts.

Duration of burn

On most lasers the laser exposure time can be varied either continuously or in increments. The effect of decreasing duration is to reduce the amount of energy delivered to the eye, as the units of energy, joules, are milliwatts per unit time (fig 2.37). Conversely, increasing the time and keeping the other parameters constant will increase the amount of energy delivered to the eye. As more energy is delivered to the eye per unit time, a burn will appear larger as duration is increased. With a short exposure burn energy will be available for absorption by a chromophore such as haemoglobin in superficial retinal vessels or retinal microaneurysms.

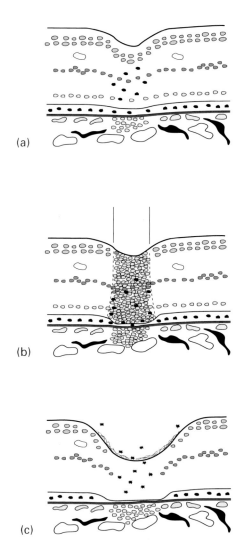

(a)

(b)

(c)

Figure 2.36 (a) Diagrammatic representation of atrophy of the retina following a laser burn with the migration of pigment cells into the retina. (b) The altered profile of the laser burn caused by absorption by the pigment cells in the retina. (c) The consequence of this burn with atrophy of the pigment epithelium, thinning of the retina, migration of pigment cells through the internal limiting membrane, and the presence of scar tissue on the surface of the retina

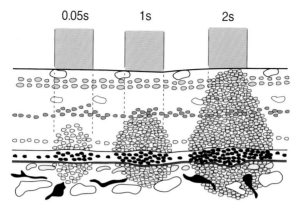

0.05s   1s   2s

Figure 2.37 Diagrammatic representation of laser burns where the power is kept constant and the exposure time is increased. The exposure time of 0·05 second produces a gentle burn on the pigment epithelium; at one second the burn is now penetrating into the more superficial retina, and at two seconds it has spread laterally and further into the retina and choroid

Number of burns

The number of burns that should be applied depends on the extent and nature of the lesions, especially in the treatment of macular oedema. In full scatter panretinal laser treatment, which requires at least 1200 burns, the use of the automatic rapid firing function will facilitate treatment, making it possible to treat large areas rapidly.

Contiguity

In full scatter panretinal photocoagulation burns are spaced at spot sized intervals and, if the retinal area is about 1500 mm^2, many thousands of burns can be accommodated. For example, 4000 spots of size 500 μm would cover only about half the retina:

$$\text{Area} = 1500 \text{ mm}^2.$$

At 500 μm or 0·5 mm size: the area of each is (πr^2) and $22/7 \times r^2$ (where r is 0·25 mm) = 0·196428.

If 4000 burns were shot:

$$4000 \times 0 \cdot 196 = 785 \cdot 7 \text{ mm}^2$$
$$785 \cdot 7/1500 = 52\%.$$

During full scatter panretinal photocoagulation burns are placed spot sized diameters apart and, if there is sufficient time for heat dispersion from the intervening retina, the burns will appear as individual lesions. If burns are placed rapidly in close proximity, the intervening retina has insufficient time to cool and will therefore receive supra-threshold damage; although at the time of treatment individual burns are visible, later the surrounding area will appear larger and confluent as a result of the heat damage to the intervening retina (fig 2.38).

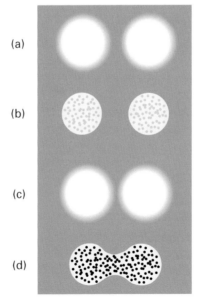

Figure 2.38 (a) The two fresh laser burns placed side by side with an interval of time between their application. This results (b) in two discrete scars on the pigment epithelium. (c) If the burns are applied more closely together in rapid succession, the effect (d) will be of a figure of eight type scar with no intervening normal retina

58

In cases with mild proliferation it will be sufficient to carry out a mild scatter panretinal treatment to arrest the proliferative activity; this consists of at least 600 burns, placed between the vascular arcades and the equator, with gaps that are much greater than a spot size diameter.

Adverse effects of laser treatment

Application of lasers may have an adverse, non-therapeutic effect on structures other than the target tissue. This damage may occur from the illuminating system, the aiming beam, or the laser beam itself. The deleterious effects are more likely in tissues that are already compromised by vascular disease and senescence.

From the slitlamp microscope

Photic damage may occur from prolonged exposure to the light of the slitlamp microscope. This damage is greatest if the light source contains blue light. The blue cones are particularly sensitive to blue light, although with most laser procedures this type of damage is unlikely to occur.

Although there have been no cases of damage caused by slitlamp microscopical examination, there is clear evidence of both transient and permanent visual loss with accompanying structural changes at the level of the RPE and photoreceptors with the operating microscope. Clearly the danger of producing damage is more likely to occur in the presence of diseased, treated, or elderly retinas but there also is an association with the duration of exposure.

To minimise the adverse effects from the illumination system the intensity should be adjusted so that the retina is adequately visualised but not excessively illuminated. Prolonged exposure to the macula should be avoided.

From the aiming beam

It has been found that the use of blue–green laser light may have a damaging effect on the observer's retina by reflection off the contact lens when the laser is not in operation. The repeated exposure results in loss of the blue cone function and there is quite marked loss after an extended treatment session, largely resolved by the following day. With repeated exposure over years there is, however, an incremental loss. This damaging effect may be prevented by avoiding the blue emission band of the argon laser. Most modern lasers now incorporate a red coaxial aiming beam and a blue–green protective filter, thus preventing damage to the operator.

Similar damage from the aiming beam may occur in the patient, particularly in one who is having multiple panretinal treatment sessions. We recommend that, when using the argon laser with the blue–green aiming beam, it should always be used on the lowest step that allows visualisation on the retina.

From the laser beam

Damage from the laser beam may occur because of unintended laser absorption, inadvertent coagulation, or scatter of the laser beam.

Unintended laser absorption

This may occur at any structure through which the laser beam passes. The degree of damage depends on the absorbing characteristics of the structure and the laser wavelength employed. Areas where absorption may occur are the edge of the iris, pigmented posterior synechiae on the lens, epicapsular stars, cortical lens opacities and nuclear xanthophyll pigment, or haemorrhages within the eye (figs 2.39 and 2.40).

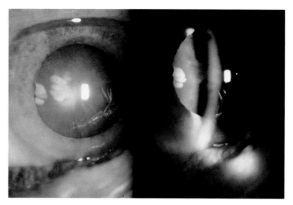

Figure 2.39 Uptake of laser at the nuclear cortex interface, in a lens with xanthophyll pigment within it. This type of lens opacity will not clear

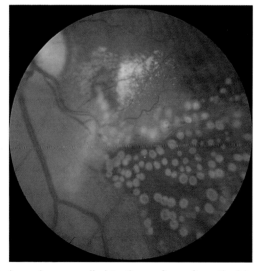

Figure 2.40 Laser burns applied to the surface of a retinal haemorrhage. This will result in uptake of heat in the nerve fibre layer and destruction of the nerve fibre and ganglion cell layers

Inadvertent coagulation

Inadvertent coagulation may occur if the wrong retinal structure is lasered. Technique is important in avoiding such

61

inadvertent coagulation of non-target structures. Photo-coagulation of the fovea may occur because of sudden ocular movement and, if cooperation is limited, a retrobulbar or peribulbar injection of an anaesthetic agent should be considered to provide akinesia (fig 2.41). The single most

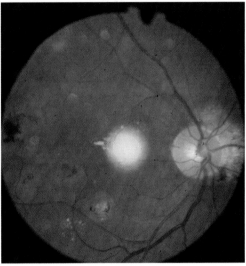

Figure 2.41 Xenon photocoagulation burn that has been inadvertently directed at the fovea

common factor associated with inadvertent lasering of the fovea is in a young patient and using the three mirror lens. Although this lens has many advantages, it is not uncommon for the operator to stray towards the posterior pole during panretinal photocoagulation. The risk is greatest when lasering the superior peripheral retina. The patient initially assists the operator by gazing upwards but, as he or she tires, the eye returns to the primary position, exposing the macula to the laser beam (fig 2.42). Knowledge of this complication can forewarn the operator and, if the three mirror lens is to be used, it is useful to demarcate the posterior retina with a ring of laser before the periphery is photocoagulated. This complication is, however, much less likely if a panfundoscopic lens is used.

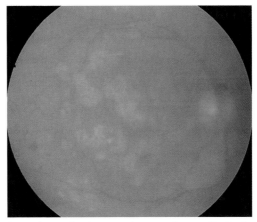

Figure 2.42   Laser burns in the macular area in a patient where the laser operator lost his way and inadvertently coagulated the macular area

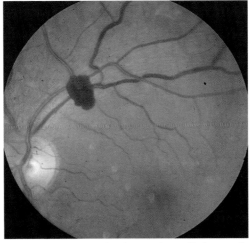

Figure 2.43   A laser burn has been inadvertently applied to a vein, resulting in occlusion of the vein and showing dilatation of the distal segment of the vein

Coagulation of the larger veins may result in spasm or temporary occlusion with obliteration of the distal segment and if new vessels elsewhere (NVE) lie on this area haemorrhage may be induced. Most often this venous

63

occlusion only lasts for a matter of hours and later fluorescein angiography usually reveals flow inside the previously lasered vessel (fig 2.43).

Scatter of the laser beam

Laser light is scattered when passing through any media opacities, and in particular vitreous haemorrhages. The longer wavelength lasers will produce less scatter than the shorter ones.

With increasing scatter of laser light, the power needed to produce a therapeutic effect at the target tissue will rise proportionally. This will also increase the likelihood of unintended collateral damage. This effect may occur if laser light is passing through thickened oedematous retina or serous elevation.

Any surface in the retina that reflects light will also produce scatter. Such surfaces are the optic disc, hard exudates, cotton wool spots, areas of retinal atrophy, previous atrophic laser scars, and fresh white laser burns. This scatter of laser off the retinal surface may account for many of the transient side effects of laser therapy, such as prolonged, reduced, visual acuity following full scatter panretinal treatment. Myopic eyes with a thin RPE or previously panretinal lasered eyes are more prone to this complication.

Non-therapeutic side effects of photocoagulation

Transient side effects

- Blurring of vision
- Choroidal detachment
- Macular oedema
- Interruption of axoplasmic flow
- Headache

Blurring of vision

Blurring of vision may be caused by persistent effects of medically induced mydriasis, anterior chamber activity as a result of released pigment, or an inflammatory response from repeated inadvertent damage to the iris.

Choroidal detachment

A peripheral choroidal detachment accompanied by a myopic shift of up to 4 D, with shallowing of the anterior chamber, is a well recognised complication of extensive dose, full scatter panretinal photocoagulation. Its importance is that it may precipitate an acute glaucoma in a patient with a pre-existing shallow anterior chamber angle. The choroidal detachment usually lasts for only 10 days and the refraction returns to pre-treatment levels. The acute glaucoma responds to acetazolamide and steroids and rarely is there a need for surgical interference (figs 2.44–2.46).

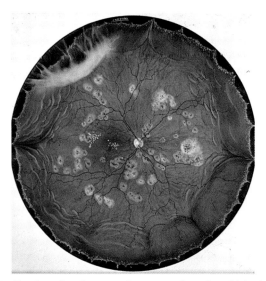

Figure 2.44 Fundus drawing to show annular choroidal detachment following xenon arc photocoagulation

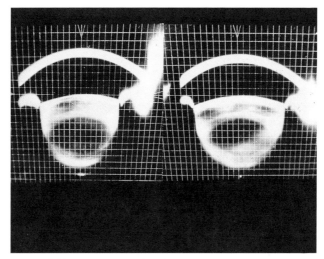

Figure 2.45 Slitlamp photograph of cornea, anterior chamber, and lens. Shallowing of the anterior chamber following panretinal photocoagulation: pre-treatment picture (above) and shallowing demonstrated on grid (below)

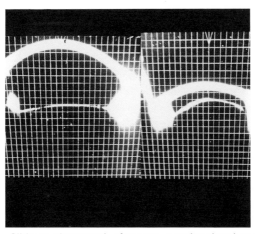

Figure 2.46 Slitlamp photograph of cornea, anterior chamber, and anterior vitreous face. Shallowing of the anterior chamber following panretinal photocoagulation in an aphakic eye, demonstrating that the effect is not caused by swelling within the lens

Macular oedema

Laser burns disrupt the blood–retina barrier and this allows fluid to leak from the choroid into the sensory retina; there the fluid may reach into the fovea along the nerve fibres. If laser is applied to the parafoveal region or to large areas beyond the vascular arcades in a full scatter panretinal pattern, this will result in a macular oedema with possible accompanying loss of visual acuity. The blood–retina barrier is restored in about 7–10 days after laser treatment and, in patients with juvenile onset diabetes, the macular oedema and visual acuity are likely to improve within four weeks. In type II diabetes, especially in patients with pre-existing macular oedema, panretinal photocoagulation may result in irreversible visual loss as a result of increased and persistent macular oedema. This deleterious effect in maturity onset diabetes is thought to be caused by age related changes such as lipid deposits in Bruch's membrane and degeneration of the RPE which is incapable of pumping the fluid towards the choroid. This mechanism is the reason why an indication for panretinal photocoagulation in the elderly patient should be made very carefully.

Interruption of axoplasmic flow

If direct laser treatment is applied to a retinal microaneurysm, using a laser wavelength that is absorbed by haemoglobin, the heat uptake from the retinal micro-aneurysm spreads horizontally to the surrounding nerve fibre layer. This can be seen as accumulation of white axoplasm on either side of the coagulated microaneurysm, and may result in some temporary visual loss, caused by conduction loss in the nerve fibre layer.

Headache

Many patients complain of headache after laser therapy. The headache may be dull and throbbing and can sometimes be accompanied by a feeling of lightheadedness and disorientation. The cause of the headache is obscure and may be the result of the lasering or the patient's anxiety associated with the laser procedure. It is generally relieved with rest and simple analgesics. It rarely persists beyond 24 hours. If the headache is severe or persistent, the patient should be assessed for angle closure glaucoma which may have been precipitated by pupillary dilatation or shallowing of the anterior chamber following photocoagulation.

Medium term side effects

Macular oedema

As mentioned above, panretinal full scatter photo-coagulation is occasionally complicated by diffuse macular oedema. Even in type I diabetes this may persist for up to three months and result in significant loss of visual acuity. Visual acuity may drop to counting fingers but the severity does not correlate with the final outcome. In type I diabetes recovery is the rule, with the vast majority eventually returning to pre-treatment visual acuity, whereas with type II diabetes the macular oedema may persist and lead to constant poor visual acuity. This complication is more common in patients with pre-existing maculopathy, and if panretinal treatment has been full scatter. Re-treating over previously treated areas of retina may also precipitate this effect.

In our experience, persistent macular oedema as a side effect of full scatter panretinal laser treatment is uncommon in young patients with previously untreated proliferative retinopathy.

In type II diabetes in those with pre-existing macular oedema, however, panretinal treatment may result in rapid irreversible progression of the maculopathy. Thus the decision for panretinal scatter treatment in elderly patients should be limited to those cases with more severe proliferation. In these patients it is important either to treat the macular oedema first and delay the panretinal treatment or to treat the macula at the same time as the panretinal photocoagulation. More rarely macular oedema may occur in type I diabetes with proliferative disease. In contrast to the ETDRS (Early Treatment Diabetic Retinopathy Study), we perform panretinal photocoagulation in this group of patients first and treat the macula later, if necessary, because in some of these young patients the macular oedema will regress spontaneously following the panretinal photocoagulation.

Persistent side effects

- Loss of visual acuity
- Accommodative defects
- Dimness
- Nyctalopia
- Loss of colour vision
- Photophobia
- Loss of visual field

Persistent side effects are not uncommon, but do vary in severity and appear to depend on the extent and intensity of the laser therapy. These side effects have a tendency to improve over months or years, although it is rare to observe a full recovery. It may be that with time the patients may adapt to the damage and become increasingly less aware of it.

Loss of visual acuity

Following full scatter panretinal photocoagulation, a small proportion of patients lose one line or more of visual acuity. The mechanism of action for this is not clear and it may well be the result of photochemical damage to the macula, possibly caused by reflected light from the peripherally placed burns. Usually there is no evidence of macular oedema. Not infrequently, this symptom is accompanied by micropsia which may indicate some anatomical derangement at the level of the photoreceptors. In some patients, improvement in visual acuity may occur over a period of 18 months.

Accommodative defects

Some patients complain of reduced near vision. In most cases this is secondary to failure of accommodation. Photocoagulation in the horizontal meridians can produce sufficient heat to damage the long ciliary nerves and cause recession of the near point. These patients inevitably need reading spectacles.

Dimness of vision

Dimness of vision is another common problem reported following full scatter panretinal photocoagulation. Some patients liken this symptom to wearing sunglasses permanently. Dimness of vision is usually dose related, and is rare in patients who have had less than 2000 exposures.

Nyctalopia

It is not surprising that some patients complain of poor night vision after full scatter panretinal photocoagulation. One might expect that, if large areas of the peripheral retina are treated, there would be a reduction in the number of rod photoreceptors with increasing scotopic thresholds. It appears, however, that reduction in photoreceptor numbers is insufficient to explain this loss fully. Furthermore, these patients also report prolonged adaptation times, with changing luminances, suggesting that other mechanisms are involved. Both symptoms appear worse in eyes that have been treated with longer duration burns (0·2 s as opposed to 0·1 s). The reason for this is equally obscure.

Colour vision

Untreated diabetic patients with diabetic retinopathy are found to have poor colour vision. This may involve all the axes with general loss of hue discrimination or just the triton axis. Following full scatter panretinal treatment, the loss becomes more pronounced, although there may be some recovery in the long term. The mechanism for this loss is not certain and may relate to direct cone destruction or be a secondary effect from scatter or damage to the blue cone nerve fibre as a result of peripheral laser treatment. The wavelength of the laser used does appear to alter this effect. A recent study has shown a tendency for near infrared diode laser panretinal treatment to cause slightly less loss of colour contrast sensitivity than argon laser panretinal photocoagulation. Also duration of burn and intensity appear to be associated with this loss.

Photophobia

The symptom of glare or dazzle is another dose related phenomenon and is more pronounced in those patients who have fair skin and those with posterior subcapsular cataracts. Glare and dazzle are almost certainly the result of hallation, that is, the scatter of intraocular light off a reflective surface. This occurs following full scatter panretinal photocoagulation when large areas of the posterior segment are devoid of normal RPE, and light is internally reflected off the bright retinal scars. The patients find their symptoms are reduced by shading their eyes, and for this reason brimmed hats or baseball caps are recommended. Sunglasses rarely help; this protection will only further dim the vision.

Loss of visual field

Field loss may occur with full scatter panretinal photocoagulation, and is greatest the more confluent the laser scars (fig 2.47). The extent of loss also depends on the number

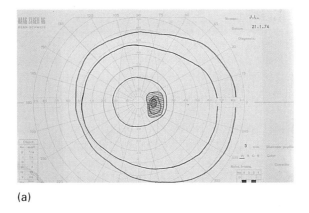

(a)

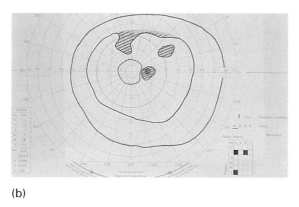

(b)

Figure 2.47 The visual field loss associated with 2000 500 μm gentle panretinal photocoagulation burns. Visual field (a) before and (b) one month later

and intensity of burns. Even a full scatter panretinal photocoagulation with threshold burns will rarely produce any loss of field, but with subsequent "fill in" the visual field will gradually deteriorate. Heavy burns or repeated treatment over the same area will result in a negative scotoma and possibly an arcuate visual field defect. Threshold burns to the posterior pole may result in small scotomata which usually fade with time. Patients after grid treatment for diffuse macular oedema will often complain of seeing a grid pattern in bright light against a light background, or transiently on blinking.

Complications of laser treatment

Complications from laser therapy do not occur only in the patient but can also occur in the laser operator. With care and skill these can be reduced, and only the most common complications will be discussed here.

Risk to the patient

Anaesthesia

Topical anaesthesia is relatively free from adverse effects, but the patient should be warned that the cornea is anaesthetised, and care should be taken to avoid injury to the eye. The risks and complications of peribulbar or retrobulbar anaesthesia are well described and include orbital haemorrhage, globe penetration, and respiratory and cardiac arrest. These risks can be reduced with careful technique and using "non-sharp" needles. The availability of resuscitation equipment is, however, mandatory if this form of anaesthesia is to be used.

Anterior segment complications

Rarely, during laser treatment for diabetic retinopathy, burns occur in the cornea and lens (fig 2.48). Both may result from defocusing the laser or from impurities on the surface of the contact lens or in the coupling fluid. The crystalline lens is more at risk from being photocoagulated if it is brunescent or has cortical opacities.

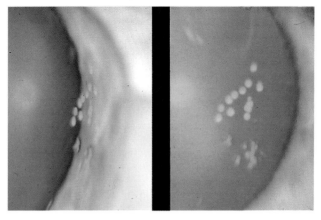

Figure 2.48   Burns in the corneal epithelium: these do not give rise to any symptoms and resolve quickly over a 24 hour period

Iritis may occur after laser therapy and, although it is mild and transient, may require topical steroids for two or three days. Iritis usually results from inadvertent lasering of the pupil margin, commonly following treatment of the peripheral retina. Sometimes iritis may follow "fill in" panretinal treatment in an eye that aready has had full scatter panretinal laser photocoagulation, even in the absence of striking the iris. The mechanism of action producing this mild anterior uveitis is unknown.

Raised intraocular pressure

Although there are a large number of causes (box D) that may produce a rise in intraocular pressure following retinal photocoagulation, the percentage of cases where a significant rise in pressure is recorded is small. In most cases in which treatment is required, the management is the same as for the non-diabetic population.

**Box D   Causes of raised intraocular
pressure following laser treatment**

- Angle closure glaucoma caused by
  choroidal detachment—postlaser
  uveitis
- Pigment dispersion
- Steroid induced glaucoma
- Rubeosis iridis

Posterior vitreous detachment   Following panretinal
laser treatment, it is not uncommon for the posterior hyaloid
face to undergo complete or partial detachment (fig 2.49).
In most cases this is benign or even advantageous, but
the possibility of causing a retinal tear should always be
considered, especially in those patients who present with
photopsia and floaters. These symptoms may not always
result from the evolving retinal scar. Rarely, detachment
of the posterior hyaloid face may elevate retinal surface
new vessels with subsequent haemorrhage or tractional
detachment of the retina. If this is away from the macula
there is no need for further treatment. By contrast, if an eye
with high risk proliferative diabetic retinopathy develops
a retinal break that results in a combined tractional and
rhegmatogenous retinal detachment, this is one of the most
complicated situations urgently requiring vitrectomy.

Heavy full thickness retinal burns should always be avoided
for the many reasons already listed. Heavy burns may produce
epiretinal membrane formation and lead to macular
puckering (fig 2.50).

Retinal complications   Inadvertent lasering of non-
target structures, especially to the fovea, is a recognised risk
of photocoagulation. To minimise this risk, care should be
taken to identify clearly all target and non-target areas before

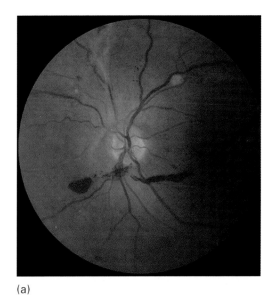

(a)

(b)

Figure 2.49 Contraction of the posterior vitreous face after panretinal photocoagulation. (a) Before treatment; (b) after treatment

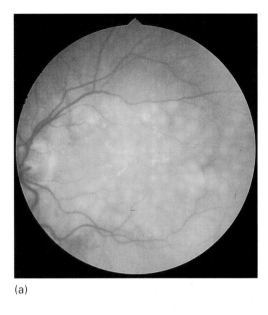

(a)

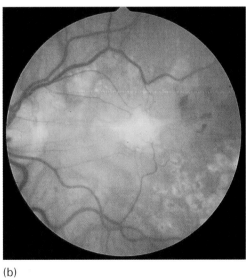

(b)

Figure 2.50 (a) Before krypton red grid treatment to the macula; (b) the development of preretinal membrane

lasering. In patients who cannot avoid ocular movement, and those requiring parafoveal treatment, short duration burns with small spot size and low powers can lower the risk to central vision. Excessive power can also result in retinal, subretinal, and choroidal haemorrhage. Rupture of Bruch's membrane may occur, resulting in choroidal neovascularisation (fig 2.51). Subretinal haemorrhages are more

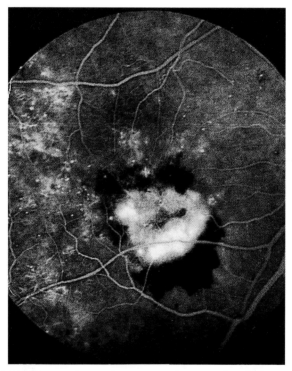

Figure 2.51 Fluorescein angiogram to show a choroidal neovascular membrane in a patient who received inadvertent high power burns to the paramacular aneurysms. This occurred as a result of failure to reduce the power, and therefore the energy density, when changing from a 500 μm burn to a 100 μm burn when approaching the macular area

common with longer wavelength lasers, because these lasers are more prone to rupture Bruch's membrane. The uptake of laser energy is more variable at longer wavelengths, and small changes in melanin density can alter the intensity of a burn considerably. Therefore the risk of haemorrhages is more common with the longer wavelength lasers. The risk of haemorrhage can be reduced by careful monitoring of the intensity of the burn. Should a haemorrhage occur, the flow can usually be stopped by gently pushing on the eye with the contact lens, to raise the intraocular pressure. Alternatively, the site of haemorrhage can be directly coagulated with a short wavelength light, such as with the blue–green laser.

Haemorrhage may also occur during attempted direct closure of retinal new vessels. Techniques to avoid this particular complication are discussed in the management of proliferative retinopathy.

Precipitation of hard exudates Sometimes when treating diabetic macular oedema, precipitation of intraretinal hard exudates may increase in the first instance following treatment. This increase in visible hard exudate may occur within one week of treatment (fig 2.52). If it occurs in the foveolar area, there may be profound loss of visual acuity. This precipitation occurs because of reduction of leakage from the retinal capillaries and microaneurysms, and so a reduction of bulk fluid flow in the retina results, leading to further deposition of lipids and proteins in the sensory retina. With the reabsorption of fluid the lipid and protein remain, and no longer flow towards the margin of the oedematous area where they are usually reabsorbed by the adjacent intact capillaries. To overcome this problem, if there are hard exudates immediately adjacent to the fovea, the focal treatment should be fractionated over weeks to months. Precipitation of hard exudates sometimes occurs after grid treatment for diffuse macular oedema and, if it does, it usually accumulates in the fovea resulting in further loss of visual acuity.

Enlargement of burns Following retinal photoco-agulation treatment, the atrophic area demarcating the original RPE burn may enlarge slowly. This delayed reaction appears to result from photochemical and photoirradiation

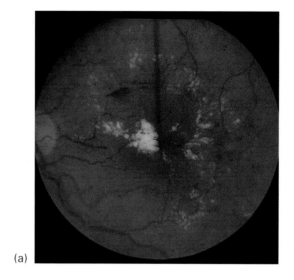

(a)

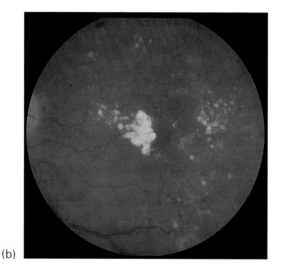

(b)

Figure 2.52 (a) Pre-treatment picture of a patient with hard exudates close to the fovea. The visual acuity was 6/12. (b) Following the laser treatment the exudates increased and the visual acuity was reduced to counting fingers. (c) Most of the exudates have absorbed, but because of the structural damage to the retina, the visual acuity did not improve

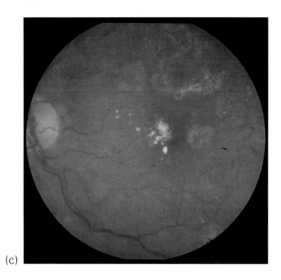

(c)

injury, sustained during laser therapy, and is localised to those RPE cells adjacent to the targeted areas (fig 2.53). The extension of the atrophic area is not normally significant unless the atrophy spreads to involve the fovea. This is unlikely unless heavy burns have been placed close to the fovea.

Choroidal neovascularisation This is an uncommon complication and usually results from high energy burns of small spot size. It is more commonly seen if long wavelength lasers have been used (see fig 2.51).

Risk to the operator

Accidental exposure

Accidental exposure to the operator of reflected laser light is uncommon, and results in the main from failure of the mechanical shutter flap. The laser operator should

81

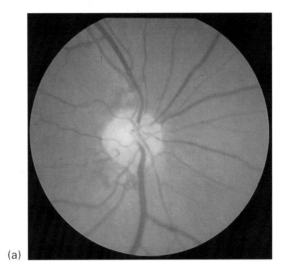

(a)

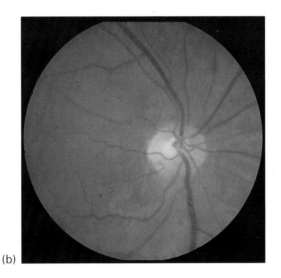

(b)

Figure 2.53 (a) Pre-treatment picture, (b) gentle burns, and (c) six months later, with enlargement and more pigmentation in the burns. This is particularly obvious in those burns immediately below the optic disc

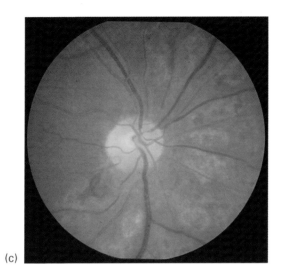

(c)

discontinue treatment immediately, if during firing the laser he or she is aware of bright "extraneous" light. The risk of this complication can be prevented by incorporating fixed protective filters. The operator may also lose blue colour vision if repeatedly exposed to reflected blue laser light coming off the aiming beam and being reflected from the contact lens.

Risk to the observer

It is not uncommon to see observers or relatives in active laser rooms. It is possible to receive sufficient energy reflected off the surface of the contact lens to cause damage, even though the beam is divergent. It has been shown that, at a distance greater than 1 metre behind the operator, it is unlikely that the divergent beam will produce a threshold burn in the observer's eye. It is, however, advised that anyone in the laser room should wear the appropriate protective goggles. In addition, all laser rooms should have an illuminated sign at the entry to indicate that a laser is in operation.

Preparation of the patient and technique of laser application

Preparation of the patient

Before laser therapy, the patient should be fully informed as to the goals of treatment and the method of delivery. If lasering in close proximity to the fovea is necessary it is important to instruct the patient to look straight ahead and to avoid any eye movements. Fixation with the fellow eye may help in these situations. It is important to discuss what is involved in laser therapy: the application of eye drops, the use of the contact lens, and the effect of laser, including non-therapeutic side effects and potential complications. Once these have been explained, the patient has to sign informed consent.

The best corrected visual acuity and immediate pre-treatment retinal findings should be recorded before therapy. We have found adequate mydriasis is usually achieved with cyclopentolate 1% or tropicamide 1% eye drops together with phenylephrine 10%. In patients with heart disease we prefer phenylephrine 2·5% as it has a lesser sympathetic effect.

Anaesthesia

Most patients usually only need topical anaesthesia to facilitate the application of a contact lens. Topical anaesthesia is not required for non-contact lens laser therapy using the indirect laser ophthalmoscope. Some patients do experience pain during laser treatment, especially during prolonged panretinal treatment sessions, if high powers are needed in eyes that are mildly pigmented, or retreating in a "fill in" pattern. Pain may also be a problem using long wavelength lasers such as the diode laser and treating beyond the vascular arcades. Pain is most frequently felt when treating in the 3, 6, 9, and 12 o'clock meridians. In these cases retrobulbar or peribulbar anaesthesia may be considered. Another possible alternative is dihydrocodeine (DF 118) tablets. This tablet, taken orally about one hour before treatment, provides adequate analgesia in many cases.

A retrobulbar or peribulbar injection of a local anaesthetic has the advantage of providing anaesthesia as well as akinesia, and this is useful in nervous patients when lasering close to the fovea.

General anaesthesia is rarely required except in very uncooperative or mentally handicapped patients, or in those with a very low pain threshold.

Contact lenses

There are a number of contact lenses used to visualise the retina during laser photocoagulation (fig 2.54). The following are the ones in common usage:

- Fundus contact lens
- Three and four mirror contact lens
- Various panfundoscopic lenses.

Fundus contact lens

This contact lens visualises the posterior pole and is an appropriate lens for treating macular lesions. An advantage is that the retinal image is not transposed.

Three and four mirror contact lens

The Goldmann mirror lenses consist of a central aperture and either three or four mirrors angled respectively to provide visualisation of the post-equatorial fundus, the equatorial fundus, and the anterior fundus. The additional mirror in the four mirror lens allows an additional view of the anterior retina. Unlike the retinal image through the central portion of the lens, which is upright, the image through the mirrors is inverted but not transposed. The central aperture of the lens visualises the posterior pole and is used for treating posterior pole lesions. The field of view through this part of the lens is

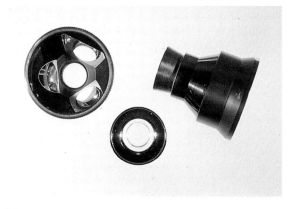

(a)

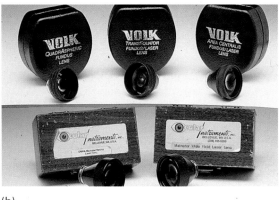

(b)

Figure 2.54   (a) Three mirror and fundus contact lenses, and a Rodenstock panfundoscope. (b) Variety of panfundoscopic lenses: the Volk Area Centralis, Transequator, and Quadraspheric, and the fundus Mainster lens and Mainster wide angle lens. These panfundoscopic lenses enable different parts of the eye to be examined, with different degrees of magnification

unfortunately smaller than through the fundus contact lens. This lens has probably been the most commonly used lens in treating diabetic retinopathy for many years. Its main disadvantage is the watershed area between the posterior pole and the largest mirror, where because of the poor view of the post-equatorial retina it is difficult to treat. This problem can be overcome if the patient is able to change his or her gaze during treatment. This will not be possible if the eye is akinetic as a result of a retrobulbar anaesthetic.

Panfundoscopic contact lenses

> - Rodenstock panfundoscope
> - Mainster Wide Field
> - Volk Area Centralis
> - Volk Transequator
> - Volk Quadraspheric

These lenses provide a good panoramic view of the retina with a field extending from the posterior pole to the peripheral fundus. As a result of the large field of view, these lenses are ideal in those patients requiring large areas of retina to be treated. Minimal cooperation is required, as the patient does not have to shift his or her gaze to allow different areas of the retina to be treated. It is possible to reach the more peripheral retina, if necessary by either tilting the lens or getting the patient to direct gaze eccentrically.

The panfundoscopic lenses are axial lenses and are particularly useful in the presence of media opacities such as cataracts, or when troublesome reflections occur at the intraocular interfaces. The retinal image is inverted and transposed, as is the image seen with the binocular indirect ophthalmoscope. The size of the burn produced by some of these lenses is larger than that achieved by the three mirror lens for the same spot size. For example, a setting of 200 µm on the slitlamp microscope will produce a burn of 286 µm at the retina with the Rodenstock Panfundus lens. As a result of the larger spot size the power density will be lower, and this may require the power setting to be adjusted. Larger spot sizes also mean the number of burns applied for an adequate panretinal scatter photocoagulation may be apparently lower with these lenses than with a three mirror lens. In practical terms 1600 burns with the Rodenstock Panfundus lens may correspond to about 2000 burns with the three mirror lens. It is generally more painful for the patients when larger spot sizes are used and it is not uncommon for smaller spot sizes (350–400 μm) to be used so as to maintain the patient's comfort.

Table 2.2 Magnification of spot size with various commercially available contact lenses

Contact lens	Spot size on retina (μm)
Spot size selector set at 200 μm:	
Volk Area Centralis	200
Goldmann three mirror	216
Volk Transequator	286
Rodenstock Panfundus	286
Mainster Wide Field	294
Volk Quadraspheric	400

Non-contact lens laser therapy

The development of the 60, 78, 90 D lenses, and Volk Superfield NC non-contact lenses, has altered not only binocular examination of the retina at the slitlamp microscope, but has also allowed for non-contact lens delivery of laser. These lenses can be fixed at the slitlamp microscope with a special device and are particularly useful in treating peripheral lesions and may be used for early treatment after cataract surgery. With modern small incision techniques, however, the operated eyes are very stable in the early postoperative period, so applying a contact lens is no longer a problem during the first days after cataract surgery.

Problems in laser treatment

In spite of the number of different lasers and the variety of contact lenses available, some problems persist that make laser treatment difficult. Some of these relate to the clarity of the media and poor visualisation of the retina, whereas others are common to procedures performed on patients in any clinic and in any hospital.

Anxiety

Many patients are nervous and apprehensive before laser therapy. This may arise because it is the first time that the patient has been treated or because of a problem occurring during previous laser sessions. Many of the patient's fears and worries can be alleviated by establishing a good rapport and an explanation of the goals of treatment. Patients will also be reassured if treatment goals are being achieved. On occasion, patients are so distraught that tranquillisers may be needed and, if the patient's anxiety reaches this level, the family practitioner must be consulted.

Pain

Pain is frequently mentioned as the main cause of anxiety for patients attending a hospital for any treatment. The pain associated with a laser is usually a sharp stabbing pain at the time of the laser application. Pain is rarely felt when treating the posterior pole but becomes more common the further anterior the laser is applied, and the areas of the 3, 6, 9, and 12 o'clock meridians anterior to the equator are the most sensitive. Pain is more with the longer laser wavelengths. Adequate analgesia should be offered to patients attending for laser treatment although this need not necessarily involve a retrobulbar or peribulbar anaesthetic. An analgesic such as a dihydrocodeine tablet one hour before treatment may be sufficient for those patients who find the laser treatment very uncomfortable. In some patients retrobulbar or peribulbar anaesthesia is required, but only rarely is a general anaesthetic required using the indirect laser ophthalmoscope. Pain is more common in lightly pigmented eyes or when treating in previously treated areas ("fill in") and in general is related to the intensity of the laser burn. Intermittent sharp stabbing pain may occur from time to time subsequent to laser therapy. This may continue for months to years after the original treatment. The cause of this is unknown.

Small pupil

Small pupils, particularly in the presence of lens opacities, can make photocoagulation treatment difficult. Some of these difficulties can be overcome by using axial contact lenses, such as panfundoscopic lenses. On occasions we have found that the 90 D non-contact lens has a role in visualising the fundus during laser treatment. On occasion, it may be necessary to revert to surgical means to enlarge the pupil.

Cataract

The presence of a cataract can interfere with laser treatment, although certain techniques may allow adequate treatment to be applied. An axial contact lens to visualise the fundus is usually best in these patients as the reflections from the opacities are minimised. A longer wavelength laser will also facilitate treatment and minimise uptake in the lens.

In some patients where the lens opacity is so dense as to preclude photocoagulation a cataract extraction should be considered with immediate laser treatment following surgery. We do not advocate "blind" cryotherapy in these patients if there is a reasonable chance of a successful cataract extraction. If trans-scleral laser treatment is needed the diode laser applied via a direct probe would be a viable treatment alternative.

Extracapsular or phacoemulsification, including a small incision technique such as a tunnel or a clear cornea incision, is the preferred method in diabetic subjects with cataracts. A posterior chamber lens is inserted into the capsular bag at the time of surgery. Foldable silicone lenses should be avoided, because a future vitrectomy and a silicone oil tamponade may be compromised.

If the eye is known to have proliferative retinopathy or macular oedema, laser treatment has to be performed within days of cataract surgery, otherwise severe deterioration of the retina may occur. Alternatively a combined cataract extraction and vitrectomy with endolaser application may be performed. In eyes where the fundus cannot be viewed preoperatively, ultrasonic examination should be performed to rule out retinal detachment. A combination of retinal detachment and cataract would also entail a combined approach.

In those eyes with active proliferative disease, intra-operative examination of the fundus with the indirect ophthalmoscope can be advised, and laser treatment can be applied via the indirect ophthalmoscope following removal of the lens and before insertion of the posterior chamber lens implant.

Myopia

Myopic eyes frequently have a very thin RPE and in these patients the choroidal vessels are often prominent. This can lead to difficulties in distinguishing between preretinal new vessels and choroidal vessels. We find, in these cases, that it is useful to perform fluorescein angiography as an adjunct to regular ophthalmoscopy.

When lasering myopic patients high energy densities are usually needed to obtain a therapeutic burn. In these eyes most of the uptake of energy occurs in the choroidal melanocytes and there is an increased risk of haemorrhage and accompanying pain to the patient.

Obesity

The obese patient is often difficult to laser because of the limitations of patient access relative to the slitlamp microscope and laser. This is especially true in treating obese women with a large bust. There is no one ideal position to laser these patients and a combination of different lenses and positions together with a lot of patience may overcome the problem. On some occasions we have found it best to lower the slitlamp microscope to the lowest limit and then move the patient stool as far from the laser as possible, so that the patient is positioned at an oblique angle leaning forward. This position will reduce the restriction of movement of the slitlamp microscope by the bust, but is usually limited by the obese abdomen which inhibits flexion of the trunk. Alternatively, the laser indirect ophthalmoscope may be helpful.

Postlaser management

In most patients, there is no necessity for any particular treatment to the eye following laser therapy. Warn patients about the problems of having an anaesthetic cornea, particularly if they have had a retrobulbar anaesthetic. It is not necessary to prescribe antibiotic ointment or eye pads unless there is evidence of corneal epithelium derangement.

Patients are also reminded of the side effects of lasering and to seek help if the eye becomes red or painful.

Laser treatment after fluorescein angiography

Argon laser will excite fluorescence and, if the laser is applied soon after fluorescein angiography, the laser flash will reflect from the eye. This will result in bleaching of the operator's visual pigments and cause temporary central scotoma making further lasering very difficult. Also the retinal effects in the patient's eye are enhanced. Thus, it is best to wait for 24 hours after fluorescein angiography before carrying out laser treatment with the argon blue–green or green laser.

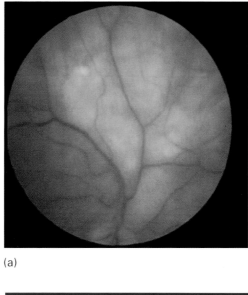

(a)

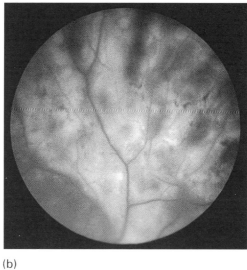

(b)

Figure 2.55   (a) Retina showing a fresh laser burn; (b) fluorescein angiogram showing leakage at the site of the laser burns

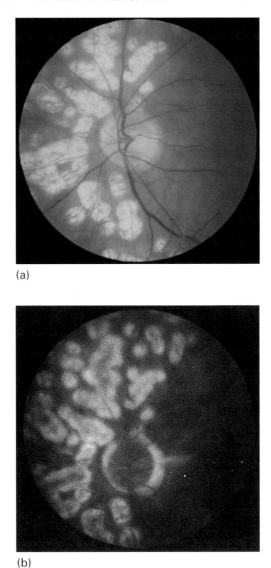

(a)

(b)

Figure 2.56   (a) Retina showing an old laser burn with hyperfluorescence and the ring of increased fluorescence at the margin of the burn; (b) fluorescein angiogram

Fluorescein angiographic appearance of the laser burn

Immediately following a therapeutic burn to the RPE the outer blood–retina barrier is disrupted and the integrity of this barrier is not restored for about 7–10 days, through a combination of cellular proliferation and migration. If fluorescein angiography is performed within 10 days of treatment a large amount of "fluorescein noise" may be seen making the angiogram difficult to interpret (fig 2.55). Once the barrier has been restored the problem ceases and only thin hyperfluorescent halos surround the burn. This halo is somewhat different depending on the laser wavelength employed, that is, with the near infrared diode laser this halo is less. This effect may be related to the lesser damage of the RPE (fig 2.56).

If large amounts of laser have been applied and there is confluence of chorioretinal atrophy late scleral staining will denote the area of burn.

3 Lesions of diabetic retinopathy

The pathogenesis of diabetic non-proliferative retinopathy consists of structural changes in the retinal capillary wall and rheological changes resulting in the closure of capillaries and leakage from the diseased vessel wall. The structural abnormalities that develop within the retinal capillary wall include the following:

- Pericyte loss
- Loss of endothelial cells
- Basement membrane thickening
- Endothelial cell dysfunction.

All these alterations result in loss of autonomic autoregulation, regulatory function, leakage from capillaries into the extracellular space of the sensory retina, and narrowing of the lumen of the capillary. The rheological changes which may result from hyperglycaemia affect the plasma, the red blood cells, and the platelets. The plasma changes include an increase in fibrinogen, α_2-globulins, and a decrease in serum albumin levels, resulting in decrease in fibrinolysis and increased viscosity. The alterations within the red blood cells are decreased deformability and, within the platelets, an increased tendency to aggregation. The combination of the histopathological alterations and the rheological effects induces closure of the retinal capillaries. This results in thrombosis within the retinal capillaries leading to the development of areas of capillary non-perfusion.

Subsequently these areas may enlarge. In the non-insulin dependent diabetic patient occur predominantly in the posterior pole, and become associated with capillary leakage and microaneurysm formation, leading ultimately to diabetic macular oedema. In the insulin dependent diabetic patient, the changes predominantly occur in the midperipheral retina leading to ischaemia, hypoxia of the retina, the production of vasoproliferative substances, and ultimately to the development of new vessel formation. The rate at which capillary closure develops and its course are very variable but the major factor is the presence of persistent or intermittent hyperglycaemia.

Individual lesions of diabetic retinopathy

- Retinal microaneurysms
- Haemorrhages
- Cotton wool spots
- Hard exudates
- Retinal oedema
- Venous changes
- Intraretinal microvascular abnormalities (IRMA)
  Intraretinal new vessels
- Preretinal new vessels elsewhere (NVE)
- Flat disc new vessels (NVD)
- Forward disc new vessels
- Fibrous tissue
- Pigment epithelial appearance change
- White blood vessels

Retinal microaneurysms

Retinal microaneurysms are dilatations of retinal capillaries. The size of the microaneurysms may vary from 10 μm up to 100 μm. Most retinal microaneurysms will appear as red dots but sometimes they will appear as a white dot. These microaneurysms are indistinguishable from dot haemorrhages except on fluorescein angiography. It is not uncommon to find either a cap of haemorrhage or a haemorrhage associated with retinal microaneurysms; this haemorrhage partly or completely surrounds the micro-aneurysms. The degree of angiographic hyperfluor-escence of the microaneurysm and the visualisation by biomicroscopy will depend on the site and extent of the associated haemorrhage. The development of a retinal microaneurysm occurs with either pouching on the side of the capillary or looping of the capillaries with ultimate fusion of the base of the loop and dilatation of the apex of the loop (fig 3.1). On fluorescein angiography the retinal microaneurysm fills at the time of the capillary bed filling. Almost always it is possible to identify a variable area of capillary non-perfusion adjacent to the area of retinal microaneurysm formation (fig 3.2). During the later stages of fluorescein angiography there may be staining of the wall of the microaneurysm. In those cases in which the microaneurysm is larger and associated with retinal oedema there will be leakage from the wall. Most microaneurysms are found in the posterior pole and in early diabetic

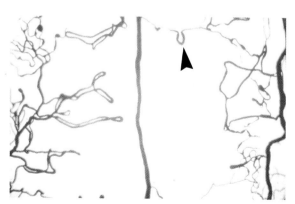

Figure 3.1   Indian ink preparation of an area of capillary non-perfusion with a developing microaneurysm seen as a loop on the retinal capillary (arrowed)

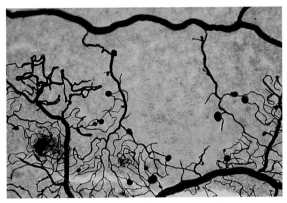

Figure 3.2   Indian ink preparation with areas of capillary non-perfusion and surrounding microaneurysms

retinopathy there is a predisposition in the area temporal to the fovea. Microaneurysms may be present in early diabetic retinopathy singly or in clumps, particularly surrounding small areas of capillary non-perfusion. The cause of microaneurysm formation is uncertain. It is possible that they represent weakening of the vessel wall in the area adjacent to capillary non-perfusion or that they may be an attempt at revascularisation of the ischaemic area. Some microaneurysms may have a cap of proliferating endothelium cells which suggests a neovascular component (fig 3.3).

Retinal microaneurysms may follow a variable course. Small microaneurysms may become larger and leak. Other retinal microaneurysms may develop a hyalinised wall and will appear white; on fluorescein angiography they may no longer be perfused. As most microaneurysms lie adjacent to an area of capillary non-perfusion, with enlargement of the area, the microaneurysms may disappear with new microaneurysms appearing later at the edge of the widening area of capillary non-perfusion. This change in micro-aneurysms with increasing non-perfusion may lead to the erroneous view that decrease in microaneurysm count has resulted in improvement of diabetic retinopathy. Although

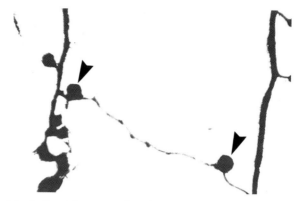

Figure 3.3   Indian ink preparation showing skeleton capillaries and other vessels full of Indian ink. Two microaneurysms can be seen (arrows) with the pale area surrounding them, indicating endothelial cell proliferation

the resolving power of the ophthalmoscope is 10 μm it is often impossible to visualise the entire population of retinal microaneurysms. With fluorescein angiography it becomes apparent that there are many more microaneurysms than are visible clinically (fig 3.4).

Haemorrhages

- Intraretinal haemorrhages
- Preretinal haemorrhages
- Vitreous haemorrhages
- Subretinal haemorrhages

Intraretinal haemorrhages

Intraretinal haemorrhages include round haemorrhages, flame shaped haemorrhages, blotch (cluster) haemorrhages, and diffuse haemorrhages.

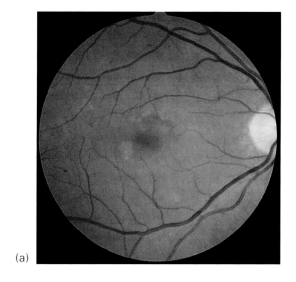

(a)

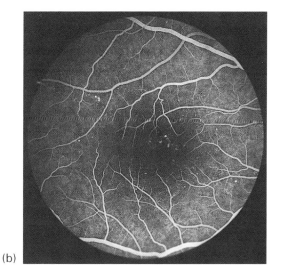

(b)

Figure 3.4 (a) Retina from a patient with diabetic retinopathy, showing a few areas of microaneurysm formation. (b) Fluorescein angiogram showing many more aneurysms than are visible in (a), showing the true severity of the retinopathy

101

Round haemorrhages

The round dot haemorrhage appears as a bright red dot the size of a large microaneurysm and rarely exceeds 200 μm in diameter. These dot haemorrhages are indistinguishable from retinal microaneurysms except on fluorescein angiography; they are always related to microaneurysms. They lie most commonly at the level of the superficial retinal capillary plexus although sometimes they lie at the level of the deep plexus. On fluorescein angiography these haemorrhages tend to block out the background choroidal fluorescence. If the haemorrhage is, however, thin then the associated microaneurysm can sometimes be identified and appears as a hyperfluorescence either in the centre of the haemorrhage or slightly eccentric to the blood. Thus the haemorrhage may lie above the microaneurysm, around the microaneurysm, partly surrounding the microaneurysm, or underneath the microaneurysm. With clearing of the haemorrhage the microaneurysm may become more visible and appear as a "normal" retinal microaneurysm, although more commonly these microaneurysms may appear pale in colour indicating a hyaline sheath or thrombosing of the microaneurysm.

Flame shaped haemorrhages

Flame shaped haemorrhages lie in the nerve fibre layer and characteristically have a filamented end oriented in the direction of the nerve fibre layer. Flame shaped haemorrhages are not uncommon in diabetic retinopathy but may also indicate associated arterial hypertension. Their extent and degree may reflect the severity of elevated blood pressure. Flame shaped haemorrhages are rarely larger than half a disc diameter in size. On fluorescein angiography they block out the background choroidal fluorescein and they obscure the capillary pattern. Flame shaped haemorrhages are most common in the area of the temporal vascular arcades and tend to be in close proximity to the optic disc (fig 3.5). Their exact cause is uncertain but it has been suggested that they result from direct pressure on the superficial capillary caused by increased arterial pressure. Flame shaped haemorrhages tend to absorb slowly but may last for a variable time—up to three months. Following absorption of the flame shaped haemorrhage fluorescein angiography will show a normal retinal capillary pattern.

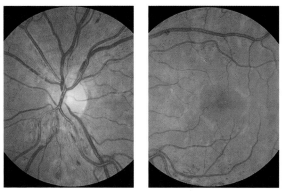

Figure 3.5 Disc and macular areas showing superficial flame shaped haemorrhages lying in the nerve fibre layer

Blotch (cluster) haemorrhages

These deep haemorrhages lie in the inner retina at the level of the outer or inner retinal capillary plexus. They have a blotchy appearance, similar to an ink blot on a pad of blotting paper. These blotch haemorrhages have a variable degree of redness depending on the extent of the oxygenation. In some areas they may appear bright red, whereas in others they appear dark. On fluorescein angiography blotch haemorrhages block out the background choroidal fluorescence and always lie either within areas of capillary non-perfusion or at the margins of capillary non-perfusion. Blotch haemorrhages are rarely single and thus they have been described as appearing in clusters. The blotch

103

haemorrhages are variable in size but are usually smaller than a quarter of a disc diameter.

Blotch haemorrhages may occur at any site in the retina, depending on the position of the capillary non-perfusion, although most commonly they are seen in the area temporal to the macula and in the area outside the central vascular arcade. The cause of blotch haemorrhages is uncertain but it is probable that they result from capillary fragility during the process of capillary closure because of their site adjacent to or in areas of non-perfusion. The evolution of blotch haemorrhages is very variable. They may take many months to resolve but in some patients, particularly if they are lying adjacent to normal capillaries, they may absorb fairly rapidly.

The presence of cluster haemorrhages is a hallmark of capillary closure and therefore an important indicator of progression of diabetic retinopathy and impending neo-vascularisation (fig 3.6).

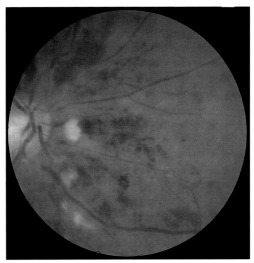

Figure 3.6 Cluster haemorrhages nasal to the optic disc indicating areas of capillary non-perfusion

Diffuse retinal haemorrhages

Diffuse haemorrhages are large haemorrhages that occupy the space between the larger retinal arterioles and venules. These haemorrhages extend throughout the full thickness of the retina, but rarely extend up to the margin of the vessel; there is therefore a haemorrhage free zone adjacent to these larger vessels. The diffuse haemorrhages are always larger than one or two disc diameters and they appear dark. They are seen in diabetic retinopathy but are much more commonly seen in other retinal vascular diseases such as central retinal vein occlusion and branch vein occlusion. On fluorescein angiography they block out the background choroidal fluorescence and are associated with capillary non-perfusion. Although at the site of haemorrhage it is not possible to see if the capillaries are non-perfused, the non-perfusion always extends up to the edge of the vessel in the area of the haemorrhage free site. These sites usually occur outside the central capillary arcade and are most commonly seen in the areas within a few disc diameters of the optic disc. Once again these diffuse haemorrhages are a feature of capillary non-perfusion and may take a considerable time, up to six months, to absorb. These haemorrhages are the precursor to the development of retinal neovascularisation—they represent capillary non-perfusion. If extensive they may also indicate impending iris neovascularisation (fig 3.7).

Petaloid haemorrhage

Another type of intraretinal haemorrhage is the petaloid haemorrhage which occurs in the equatorial region and anterior equatorial retina. These haemorrhages lie in the superficial retina and look like the chrysanthemum flower. They have peripheral streaks which extend into the superficial retina. These haemorrhages, which are variable in size and tend to vary in colour, some remaining bright red whereas others are rather dark, lie immediately underneath the internal limiting membrane. On occasion it is obvious that

105

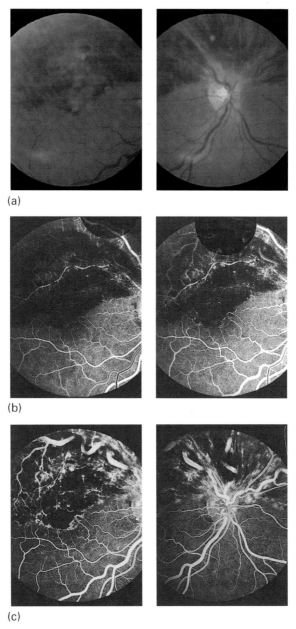

(a)

(b)

(c)

Figure 3.7 (a) Retina, and (b) early and (c) late fluorescein angiograms, showing a diffuse haemorrhage and the accompanying capillary non-perfusion

they are related to rather larger retinal microaneurysms which lie in the equatorial region of the retina. The size of these lesions varies considerably and some are small whereas others may be of a size almost up to a disc diameter. Fluorescein angiography will block out the background choroidal fluorescence at the site of these haemorrhages and it is unusual to see the accompanying microaneurysm. These haemorrhages frequently lie in areas of capillary non-perfusion (fig 3.8). The long-term significance of these haemorrhages is somewhat uncertain.

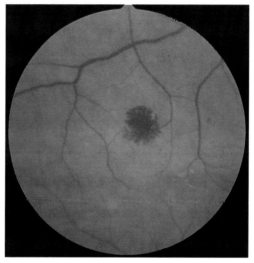

Figure 3.8   Typical retina showing a petaloid haemorrhage, seen here in the pre-equatorial area

Preretinal haemorrhages

Subinternal limiting membrane haemorrhage

These haemorrhages may occur in the macular or paramacular region. They are most commonly associated with a Valsalva manoeuvre and new vessels elsewhere (NVE) and may appear as small round localised haemorrhages (see fig 3.10) or larger boat shaped haemorrhages (fig 3.9). On fluorescein angiography this type of haemorrhage blocks out the underlying retinal vessels and capillaries. Subhyaloid haemorrhages are derived from either superficial capillaries or new vessels on the disc or elsewhere. Subhyaloid haemorrhages, which tend to absorb very slowly, may end up in epiretinal fibrous tissue formation (fig 3.9(e)). During evolution it is possible that these haemorrhages may become yellow–white which represents altered blood within the haemorrhage; on occasion it may consist of two layers with the altered haemorrhage above and the red blood below with a horizontal border between the two (fig 3.9(d)). If a large subhyaloidal haemorrhage is located in the foveal region, opening of the internal limiting membrane the Nd:YAG

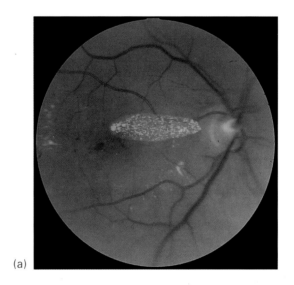

(a)

Figure 3.9 (a) Retina of a diabetic patient before development of a large subhyaloid haemorrhage; (b) immediately following the development of the subhyaloid haemorrhage, (c) slow settling of this haemorrhage, (d) a white area on top of the haemorrhage, denoting a separation of the red cells, and (e) appearance six months after the initial haemorrhage, showing a pale area denoting organised subhyaloid haemorrhage. These haemorrhages may induce preretinal fibrosis

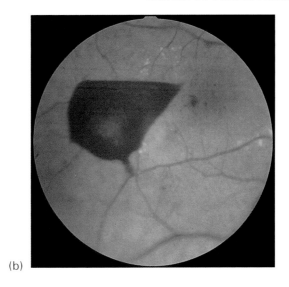

(b)

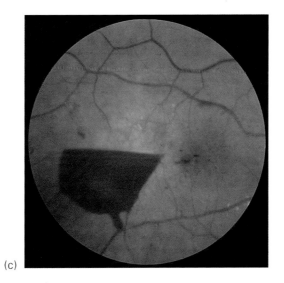

(c)

Figure 3.9   contd

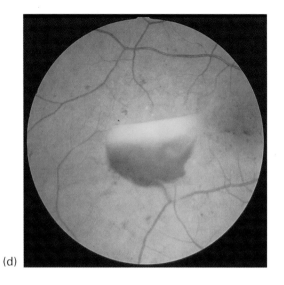

(d)

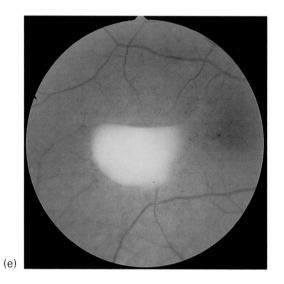

(e)

Figure 3.9   contd

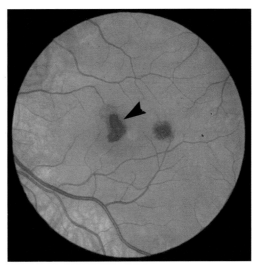

Figure 3.10 Small "round" preretinal haemorrhage (arrow) following a Valsalva manoeuvre

laser is the treatment of choice. If the resulting vitreous haze fails to clear a vitrectomy may be required. Small haemorrhages such as in fig 3.10 should not be lasered because there is a risk of creating a macular hole.

Treament of subhyaloidal haemorrhage

Extrafoveal—wait, no treatment
Prefoveal
  Small round—wait
  Large boat shaped—Nd: YAG laser

Vitreous haemorrhage

Vitreous haemorrhages result from bleeding from NVE or disc new vessels (NVD), and lie in the retrohyaloid space or, if there is sufficient force or the blood vessel is lying in the hyaloid membrane, the haemorrhage may extend into the vitreous gel itself. Therefore the site and extent of the haemorrhage may limit the view of the source of bleeding. Fluorescein angiography may identify the new vessel that has given rise to this type of haemorrhage. If the new vessel does not continue to bleed then the haemorrhage will gradually be absorbed, although the view of the retina and the patient's vision may improve earlier as a result of the haemorrhage sinking to the dependent part of the eye. Thus the patient's vision may benefit from sleeping in an erect position. The clearing of the vitreous gel will, however, depend on whether there is re-bleeding from the new vessels. In some cases the recurrent re-bleeding will prevent complete absorption and the haemorrhage persists for a long period of time. With absorption of a haemorrhage within the vitreous body, localised patches may remain particularly in the inferior part of the vitreous, and these whitish fluffy patches may persist almost indefinitely. Long standing vitreous haemorrhage may result in functional retinal damage and this could compromise the final visual outcome even after successful vitrectomy.

Cotton wool spots

Cotton wool spots are a common feature of diabetic retinopathy and appear as white fluffy opaque areas in the sensory retina. A cotton wool spot results from an arteriolar occlusion in the nerve fibre layer. This causes an accumulation of axoplasm at the site of the adjacent area of capillary non-perfusion. The axoplasm is derived from both orthograde and retrograde flow and cystoid bodies are the histological representation; cystoid bodies are macrophages filled with axoplasmic debris. The typical cotton wool spot can be seen by biomicroscopy to lie in the nerve fibre layer and is arranged in its long axis. Most cotton wool spots have a fairly uniform size, being less than half a disc diameter.

Small, superficial, flame shaped haemorrhages are often related to cotton wool spots; again these often lie along the axis of the nerve fibre layer (fig 3.11). On fluorescein angiography in the area of the cotton wool spot there is capillary non-perfusion; it is sometimes possible to identify the arteriole that has become occluded. Surrounding the area of the cotton wool spot, there is almost uniform capillary dilatation and, in addition, there may be some staining of fluorescein or even leakage of fluorescein from the surrounding dilated capillaries.

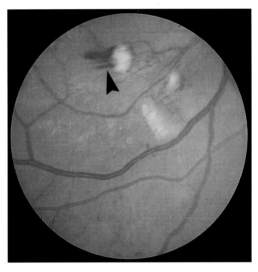

Figure 3.11   Three cotton wool spots of varying size; in one area there is, in addition, a superficial flame shaped haemorrhage (arrow)

Cotton wool spots are almost always confined to the area adjacent to the major vascular arcade. It is unusual to see them in the equatorial or pre-equatorial region. The number of cotton wool spots is very variable. In patients with progressive retinopathy there may be more cotton wool spots at various stages of development. Cotton wool spots may occur as a result of arterial hypertension which can be a common accompaniment for patients with diabetes and diabetic retinopathy. Cotton wool spots may also be present in pregnant diabetic women with progressive retinopathy. In addition, cotton wool spots are a feature of patients who have had a rapid improvement in control of previously poorly controlled diabetes.

The evolution of cotton wool spots in diabetic retinopathy is somewhat variable. Many cotton wool spots associated with diabetic retinopathy persist for three to six months as compared with those of arterial hypertension which may disappear after a period of six weeks. As cotton wool spots resolve slowly they often appear as multiple small round white dots. As these lesions disappear, the clinical appearance of the retina returns to normal. Similarly, the appearance of the fluorescein angiogram may show that the retinal capillaries reopen and return to a state of normal perfusion. If, however, the cotton wool spot lies adjacent to an area of capillary non-perfusion, there may not be reperfusion of the retinal capillaries.

Cotton wool spots represent an interruption in axoplasmic flow and they are sometimes seen adjacent to superficial laser burns. If laser is applied to superficial retinal microaneurysms and this results in uptake of heat by the microaneurysm, then within 24 hours it is possible to see fluffy accumulation of axoplasm on either side of the microaneurysm. This interruption of axoplasmic flow is short lived and will have disappeared within a week of the laser therapy. Cotton wool spots, although representing areas of capillary non-perfusion, should not be lasered. Similarly the haemorrhages that surround the cotton wool spots should be avoided and, although there may be leakage from the adjacent capillaries, this is a short lived phenomenon not requiring laser therapy. If laser is, however, applied to an area of cotton wool spot most of the laser will be reflected back from the grey–white surface and therefore fail to reach the retinal pigment epithelium (RPE). Cotton wool spots depend on the integrity of arterioles and the nerve fibre layer. If an area or areas show extensive capillary non-perfusion even in the presence of severe arterial hypertension, cotton wool spots will not form.

Retinal oedema

This can be intracellular retinal oedema (cloudy swelling) or extracellular retinal oedema.

Intracellular retinal oedema (cloudy swelling)

If the capillary non-perfusion is more widespread smaller cotton wool spots do not form. The area may, however, take on a grey–white appearance in the acute stage of closure. This appearance is often accompanied by rather fluffy small lesions which look like exudates. The grey area represents cloudy swelling of the nerve fibre layer and the ganglion cell layer accompanying the capillary non-perfusion. These changes are most common in the area surrounding the fovea, particularly in the area temporal to it. If these changes occur in the foveolar area there is often accompanying cystoid oedema and, without a fluorescein angiogram, it is impossible to distinguish this appearance from that in some of the patients with diffuse extracellular macular oedema. On fluorescein angiography the greyish area shows capillary, arteriolar, and venular occlusion (fig 3.12).

Surrounding these greyish areas there is dilatation of retinal capillaries and frequently leakage. With resolution of this greyish area there is no reperfusion and on fluorescein angiography the capillary non-perfusion persists. The loss of the grey colour in these areas may take many months and leads to atrophy of the outer layers of the retina; it may also result in some disturbance in the RPE. This type of change frequently occurs in maturity onset diabetes, particularly in those patients with arterial hypertension and arteriosclerosis. The appearance of multiple areas with fluffy type exudates in the posterior pole is very characteristic of the type change that may occur in diabetic patients with uraemia. Cloudy swelling is not an indication for focal laser treatment.

115

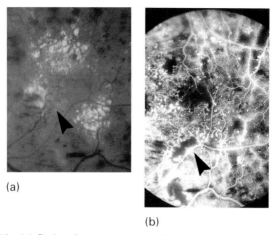

(a)

(b)

Figure 3.12 (a) Retina from a patient with mixed maculopathy, showing areas of capillary non-perfusion, leakage, and an area of resolving intracellular retinal oedema (arrow); (b) fluorescein angiogram. The area of resolving intracellular retinal oedema corresponds with the area of closure seen arrowed on the fluorescein angiogram

Extracellular retinal oedema

Extracellular retinal oedema occurs as a result of leakage from dilated capillaries and retinal microaneurysms with breakdown of the blood–retina barrier. The accumulated fluid lies in the outer plexiform layer and may either stretch or disrupt the Müller fibres running vertically in the retina (fig 3.13). If the fluid is in the foveal area it may form layer spaces of so called cystoid macular oedema.

Extracellular retinal oedema is very difficult to detect with the direct ophthalmoscope, but with high magnification stereoscopic biomicroscopy it may be seen as retinal thickening; cystoid oedema will have a petaloid appearance in the fovea with possibly some accentuation of the yellow luteal pigment xanthophyll (fig 3.14). Even with careful examination it is sometimes difficult to detect small areas of shallow thickening of the retina. On fluorescein angiography, however, leakage into the retina can be more clearly identified and during the passage of dye there is increasing accumulation of fluorescein within the sensory retina. In some patients in

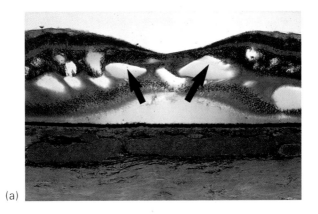

(a)

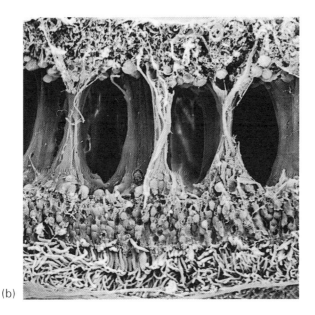

(b)

Figure 3.13 (a) Histological preparation of the retina showing fluid filled spaces (arrowed); (b) electron micrograph of cystoid spaces within the retina, showing Müller's fibres with the remaining nerve fibres pressed against the Müller's fibres; (c) electron micrograph of cystoid macular oedema in which there is not only disruption of the nerve fibre layer but also of Müller's fibres; (d) diagrammatic representation of cystoid macular oedema

117

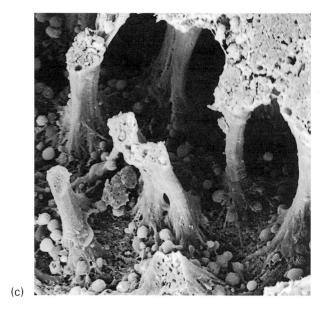

(c)

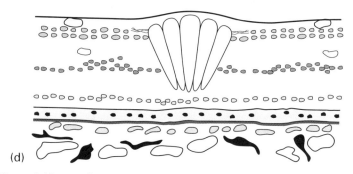

(d)

Figure 3.13   contd

the early pictures of the dye transit, leakage can be seen not only from the retinal vessels but also from the RPE—so called deep leakage. Most lesions responsible for retinal oedema lie either in the region of the superficial or deep retinal capillary plexus (fig 3.15).

118

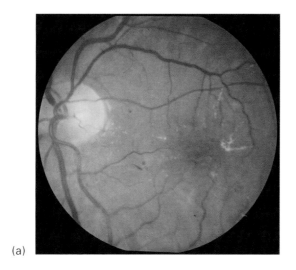

(a)

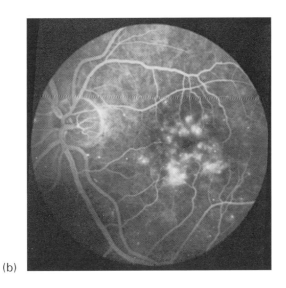

(b)

Figure 3.14 (a) Cystoid macular oedema; (b) intermediate stage on fluorescein angiogram; (c) late stage showing accumulation of the dye within the cystoid spaces in the macula

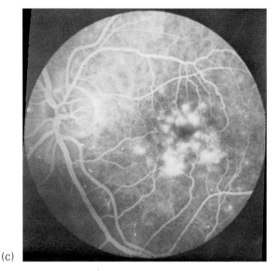

(c)

Figure 3.14   contd

The extracellular fluid in the retina is dynamic but is flowing from the area of leakage to the adjacent relatively normal capillaries where it is absorbed. If the amount of fluid is excessive it may flow in a dependent direction. The nature of the fluid will depend on the degree of breakdown of the blood–retina barrier. The greater the breakdown, the more the larger molecular weight plasma constituents, such as lipids and proteins, will pass through into the extracellular spaces. They travel with the bulk flow of the fluid to the relatively normal adjacent capillaries, where the fluid is reabsorbed and the lipid and protein are deposited. This extracellular fluid containing protein and lipid is relatively opaque and will often obscure the deeper structures such as deep plexus retinal microaneurysms; it will also contribute to scatter of laser light, so that increasing severity of cystoid oedema is associated with increasing visual loss. Retinal thickening caused by extracellular retinal oedema is a hallmark of clinically significant macular oedema which requires focal or grid laser treatment.

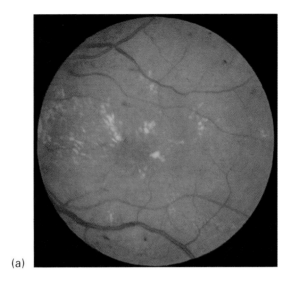

(a)

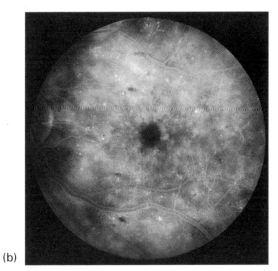

(b)

Figure 3.15   From a patient with diffuse macular oedema: (a) retina showing marked venous beading; (b) fluorescein angiogram showing areas of capillary closure

Hard exudates

- Dot hard exudates
- Fluffy hard exudates
- Plaque hard exudates

Hard exudates represent an accumulation of lipid and/or protein within the sensory retina. They have a predilection for the posterior pole and may lie both temporal and nasal to the optic disc. Hard exudates may appear in three different configurations: as dots, as fluffy hard exudates, or as more well circumscribed plaques. They can be deposited in the superficial retina, in the deeper layers of the retina, and in the macula in the nerve fibre layer of Henle. Hard exudates are formed in relation to leaking capillaries and/or retinal microaneurysms. They are generally deposited in the sensory retina at the junction of abnormal and relatively normal capillaries (fig 3.16). The plaque exudate which may occur in the fovea is, however, usually surrounded by abnormal

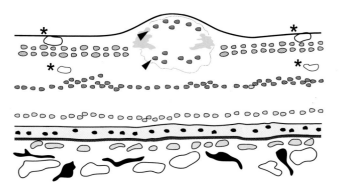

Figure 3.16 Diagrammatic representation to show leaking capillaries and microaneurysms (arrow), exudate formation surrounding this area (*), and thickening of the retina

capillaries. The clinical appearances of these three types of hard exudates are discussed below. Hard exudates are a hallmark of clinically significant macular oedema which requires focal or grid laser treatment.

Dot hard exudates

The dot hard exudates seen on biomicroscopy consist of small round yellow spots, lying superficially or deep in the sensory retina; they are about 10 μm in diameter and represent macrophages full of lipid or protein. These dots, if examined over months, will form different patterns and represent macrophages migrating through the retina (fig 3.17).

Fluffy hard exudates

The fluffy hard exudates, which are often associated with resolving cloudy swelling of the retina, appear as paler yellow deposits which tend to lie more superficially in the sensory retina. These fluffy deposits may also be seen following laser treatment when fluid is being absorbed from the retina (see fig 3.12).

Plaque hard exudates

Plaque hard exudates vary in size and represent more diffuse accumulation of lipid and protein in the retina. Plaques that form in the fovea are associated with extensive leakage in the posterior pole and poor vision (fig 3.18). With progressive closure of capillaries in the posterior pole a plaque may gradually resolve leaving behind an RPE scar (fig 3.16).

Hard exudates can be arranged in different patterns. They may be circinate in pattern surrounding an area of abnormal leaking capillaries and microaneurysms (fig 3.19), or they may be scattered over the retina not taking on any particular

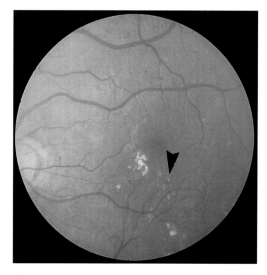

Figure 3.17   Dot exudates (arrow)

configuration (figs 3.20–3.22). If hard exudates are re-photographed over a period of time the pattern of the hard exudate may change, indicating the absorption of lipid and protein back into the retinal microcirculation. This re-absorption is caused by the activity of macrophages which migrate through the retina to the adjacent, relatively normal capillaries. Evolution of hard exudates depends on the degree and extent of the leakage and the bulk flow, in that if areas of leaking microaneurysms should resolve spontaneously, either with the microaneurysm thrombosing or with closure of the capillary supplying the microaneurysms, then the accompanying hard exudate itself may resolve. If the area of capillary closure related to the hard exudate should enlarge the exudate ring itself may enlarge. Therefore hard exudates adjacent to the fovea with increasing severity of disease may extend into the foveal area.

With decreasing leakage following focal laser treatment, plaque exudates in the fovea will slowly resolve but will leave

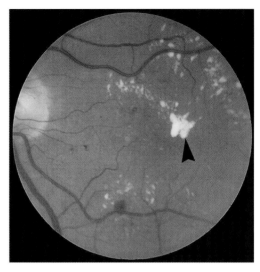

Figure 3.18   Plaque exudate (arrow)

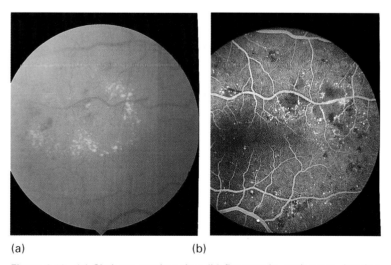

(a)   (b)

Figure 3.19   (a) Circinate exudate ring; (b) fluorescein angiogram showing areas of capillary closure with surrounding leaking microaneurysms. There is also staining and leaking from an arterial wall that is passing through the area of capillary non-perfusion

125

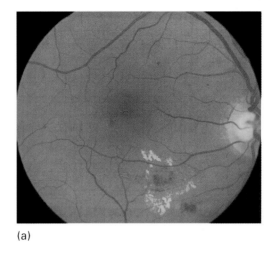

(a)

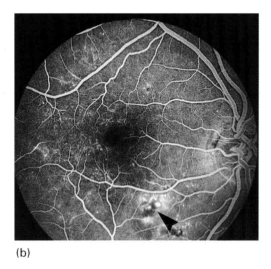

(b)

Figure 3.20 (a) Retina showing a well defined circinate exudate ring and two large microaneurysms with surrounding leaking capillaries (arrow in (b)); adjacent to the aneurysms is an area of capillary closure; (b) fluorescein angiogram

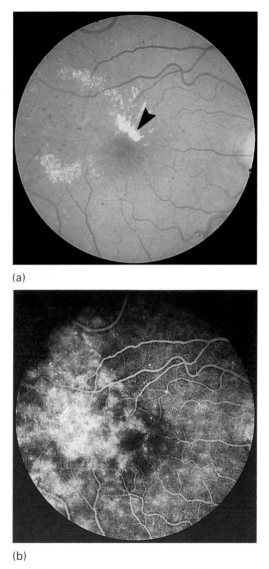

(a)

(b)

Figure 3.21   (a) A large circinate exudate ring with red dots representing aneurysms. (a) Note that the exudate ring is made up of a plaque exudate (arrow) and dot exudates; (b) fluorescein angiogram showing leakage predominantly within the circinate ring

127

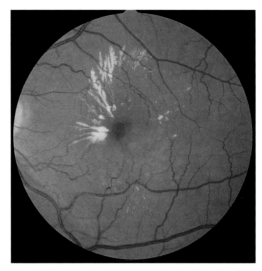

Figure 3.22   Scattered exudates with no particular configuration

behind an RPE scar with associated poor visual acuity. Hard exudates may also be present as a result of complications of other associated conditions. In diabetic subjects with arterial hypertension there may be increased leakage and so increased deposition of hard exudates. A macular star may accompany more severe arterial hypertension.

Hard exudates are also frequently present in patients with uraemia and these hard exudates may be of any type. With correction of the uraemia there may be considerable resolution of oedema and hard exudate formation. The treatment of hard exudates is indirect and related to the area of capillary or microaneurysm leakage. Laser treatment to areas of leakage may initially increase hard exudate formation because of the deposition of protein and fat in the retina, resulting from loss of bulk fluid flow through the sensory retina. If this increase in hard exudate is in the foveal region there will be accompanying loss of visual acuity (see fig 2.52).

Hard drusen which may be present in the macular and paramacular area of elderly patients can sometimes be confused with diabetic hard exudates. This confusion can be resolved by fluorescein angiography with careful examination of the stereo photographs to identify the levels of hyperfluorescence.

Venous abnormalities

- Venous dilatation
- Venous beading
- Venous loops
- IRMA

Venous dilatation

Venous dilatation is the earliest change described in diabetic retinopathy. This may be a very difficult sign to assess clinically but on occasions it is so obvious that it is easily recognised. This change represents the preclinical stage of diabetic retinopathy and may be associated with increase in blood flow through the retina.

Venous beading

Venous beading is a common accompaniment to severe non-proliferative diabetic retinopathy. Clinically this sign appears as a variable degree of sausage like dilatation and narrowing in the retinal veins. It may occur in any order of vein or venule and is associated with venous dilatation. On fluorescein angiography, there is always a degree of capillary non-perfusion in the area of venous beading. This sign is therefore a good indicator of the extent and severity of capillary closure. The changes of venous beading are more pronounced on the larger retinal veins. Eyes with venous beading need close surveillance because they are prone to proliferation (fig 3.23).

Venous loops

Venous loops are localised areas of deviation of the vein in the manner of an ox bow lake. Loops may be present on

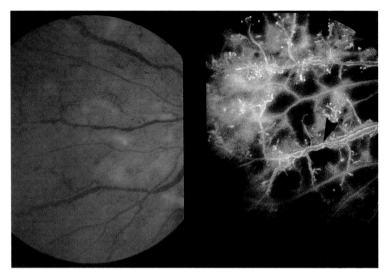

Figure 3.23 (a) Retina showing venous beading; (b) accompanying fluorescein angiogram

any order of vein or venule, but are most common on the larger veins. They form as the result of two possible mechanisms:

- With the development of collateral channels around a site of occlusion (fig 3.24). Collateral channels during the evolution of an occlusion may be numerous and multiple but may resolve into a single or double channel (fig 3.25).
- As the result of fibrous tissue occurring in the loop of a vessel, contracting and creating a loop.

Of these varieties the most common is the type in which there is occlusion of the retinal vessel. In these patients, on fluorescein angiography, the area peripheral to the loop will show capillary non-perfusion and if the disease has extended further there may also be non-perfusion proximal to the loop. The evolution of these changes is somewhat variable. They may slowly narrow and, with narrowing of the retinal vessels, they may thrombose with occlusion of the associated vessels.

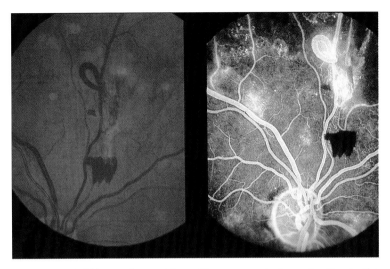

Figure 3.24 (a) Venous loop with capillary non-perfusion extending to the periphery from the area of the loop; (b) fluorescein angiogram

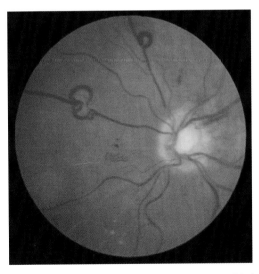

Figure 3.25 Two areas of loop formation: one shows a double loop and the other a single

Laser treatment is not indicated for these as they represent a reparative collateral channel around the areas of venous closure. Venous loops have no prognostic value for the progression of diabetic retinopathy or the development of proliferative diabetic retinopathy.

Intraretinal microvascular abnormalities (IRMA)

IRMA are defined as dilated retinal capillaries, which are often difficult to assess, and fluorescein angiography may be needed. IRMA are a hallmark of severe non-proliferative diabetic retinopathy and they are a precursor of proliferative retinopathy. Today IRMA and intraretinal new vessels are considered to be the same. By definition, intraretinal new vessels are IRMA as long as they are not breaking through the internal limiting membrane.

New vessels elsewhere

Intraretinal NVE

Intraretinal new vessels develop in areas of capillary non-perfusion. They are most commonly seen in the post-equatorial region and in the area temporal to the macula. They form as a consequence of capillary non-perfusion and most commonly develop in areas of capillary non-perfusion that are surrounded by viable perfused retina. Only rarely are they seen related to the margin of peripheral non-perfusion. The earliest sign of the development of an intraretinal new vessel is a small bud coming off a retinal vein or venule. These buds slowly extend into the non-perfused area and have an appearance like a hairpin (fig 3.26). They tend to branch and may ultimately fill the entire area of non-perfused retina. These intraretinal new vessels always develop from venous trunks. They are identifiable clinically as irregular branching of the venules and the diameter rarely exceeds 10 μm. At the growing end of the vessels, however, there may be some dilatation and sometimes

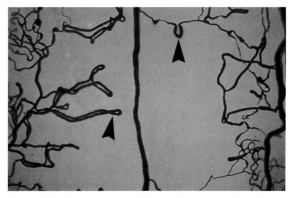

Figure 3.26   Left: Indian ink preparation to show the hairpin like intraretinal new vessels (arrow). Right: in addition in this preparation there is a loop in a capillary (arrow) representing the early development of a microaneurysm

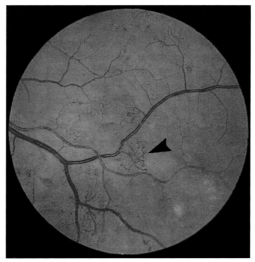

Figure 3.27   Several areas of intraretinal new vessel formation extending into an area of capillary non-perfusion with dilated growing ends (arrow)

the tip resembles a microaneurysm. On fluorescein angiography these vessels are perfused. In the later stages of the angiogram there may be some staining of the growing

133

tip. These vessels represent an attempt to reperfuse the ischaemic areas (fig 3.27).

On histological examination, intraretinal NVE have been shown to result from either recanalisation of existing basement membrane tubes, and on occasion there may be reduplication of the basement membrane suggesting vessel growth, or the growth of new capillaries into the ischaemic retina. The significance of intraretinal new vessels is that they represent intraretinal revascularisation of the retina and clinically they are a marker to areas of capillary non-perfusion.

Intraretinal NVE indicate areas where preretinal NVE may be present or anticipated. Intraretinal NVE in themselves do not therefore represent any threat to vision, and do not represent an indication for laser treatment.

Preretinal NVE

- Flat
- Forward
- Raspberry (abortive neovascular outgrowths) (ANO/NVE)
- Choroidal neovascularisation (CNV)

Preretinal NVE above the internal limiting membrane develop as the result of capillary non-perfusion and ischaemia. NVE generally occur at the margin of areas of non-perfusion but disc new vessels (NVD) will only occur if there is more than one quarter of the entire retina involved with capillary non-perfusion and ischaemia. NVE on the retina, in most cases, are derived from retinal veins but may on rare occasions develop from retinal arteries. Those derived from the arteries are more difficult to treat than the ones derived from veins.

Another source of retinal NVE is the choroid and this only occurs from sites of previous chorioretinal scarring. Retinal new vessels initially lie on the surface of the retina. They

They become attached to the posterior vitreous face and, with the passage of time, the vitreous may contract pulling the vessels off the surface of the retina. Any new vessel that forms may have accompanying adventitial scar tissue. This appears in the retina as grey–white tissue made up of collagen within the area of new vessels.

Flat retinal NVE

New vessels are derived in most cases from retinal veins. They grow out of the veins or venules and quickly penetrate through the internal limiting membrane to lie between the cleavage of the internal limiting membrane, representing the surface of the retina, and the posterior vitreous face (fig 3.28). Once a vessel has penetrated into this space, it has lost the support of the retina and is therefore prone to traction forces by the posterior vitreous face and also changes in intravascular pressure. Either of these two effects may result in a haemorrhage. These vessels may spread on the surface of the retina; the pattern of the vessels is very variable and the spread is irregular across the retina (fig 3.29). The

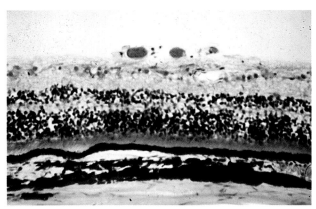

Figure 3.28 Histological preparation of the retina showing a new vessel lying on the surface of the retina, having passed through the internal limiting membrane

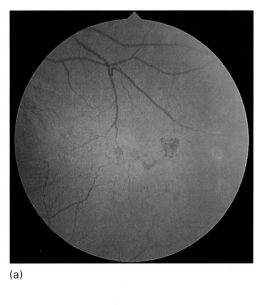

(a)

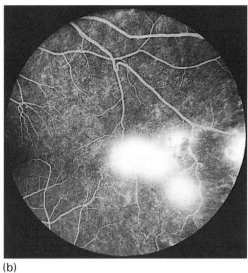

(b)

Figure 3.29 (a) Small area of new vessels adjacent to some previously applied laser treatment; (b) fluorescein angiogram showing the vessels and the adjacent non-perfusion and leakage from the vessels

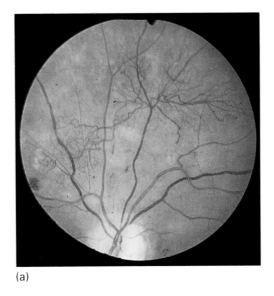

(a)

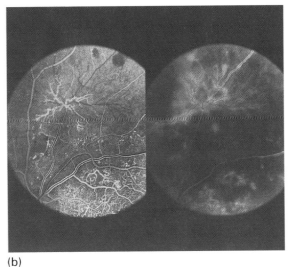

(b)

Figure 3.30 (a) A large area of new vessel formation derived from a retinal vein and draining into the same vein, and also anastomosing with a new vessel from the adjacent vein. (b) Fluorescein angiogram showing the early filling of the new vessel, the adjacent area of the capillary non-perfusion, and the late staining and leakage of the vessel

diameter of the vessels may be as great as 200–300 μm. The vessels, however, may be extremely fine, down to 10 μm, and the growing end of the vessel may be dilated. On fluorescein angiography, once the vessel has penetrated the internal limiting membrane, there is a variable degree of fluorescein leakage (fig 3.30). In some patients there is profuse leakage; in others the leakage is minimal.

Forward retinal NVE

Surface retinal new vessels may be pulled forward by the detaching vitreous face or may grow from an area of vitreous attached along the already detached vitreous (figs 3.31 and 3.32). In this situation they are prone to the influence of the mobile vitreous gel and are more likely to bleed. Only rarely do they penetrate through the posterior hyaloid membrane. With complete detachment of the vitreous, the new vessel may be avulsed from the retina and form a ghost of the vessel

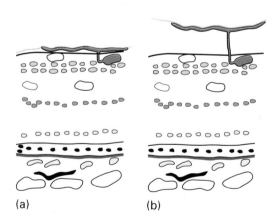

(a)   (b)

Figure 3.31 (a) Diagrammatic representation of a surface retinal new vessel with posterior vitreous face attached to the new vessel. (b) Contracted posterior vitreous face pulling the vessel off the surface of the retina

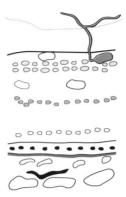

Figure 3.32   New vessel that has penetrated the posterior vitreous face to lie within the vitreous itself

on the posterior hyaloid. Forward NVE will with time be accompanied by fibrous tissue and this results in a variable degree of traction. Forward NVE tend to leak profusely on fluorescein angiography (figs 3.33 and 3.34).

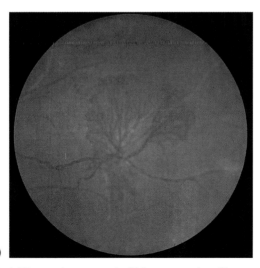

(a)

Figure 3.33   (a) Forward new vessel within an area of capillary non-perfusion; (b) fluorescein angiogram showing considerable leakage from the new vessel

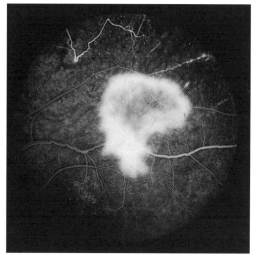

(b)

Figure 3.33   contd

"Raspberry" NVE/ANO

Abortive neovascular outgrowths (ANO) may be seen as small red patches rather like a raspberry of up to 500 µm in diameter with an intertwining vascular pattern and a central fibrous cone (figs 3.35 and 3.36). On fluorescein angiography these "raspberries" hyperfluoresce, leak profusely, and lie adjacent to areas of capillary non-perfusion. They tend to bleed fairly readily and usually lie in the area temporal to the fovea within the vascular arcades (fig 3.37).

Choroidal neovascularisation (CNV)

New vessels may be derived from the choroidal circulation in patients in whom laser or xenon light therapy has already been carried out. The previous treatment must have been heavy; associated rupture of Bruch's membrane is suspected. This CNV tends to grow from the margin of the photo-coagulation burn and may extend to the surface of the retina

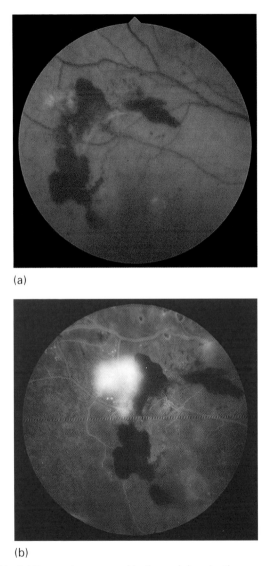

(a)

(b)

Figure 3.34   (a) Forward new vessel in the peripheral retina, associated with fibrous tissue and haemorrhage formation; (b) fluorescein angiogram

or up to the posterior vitreous face (see fig 2.51). They can be shown to be of choroidal origin in early frames of the fluorescein angiography. In the later stages of angiography

141

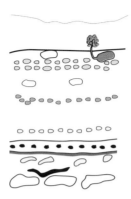

Figure 3.35   Diagrammatic representation of a "raspberry;" there is a small fibrous core with surrounding vessels

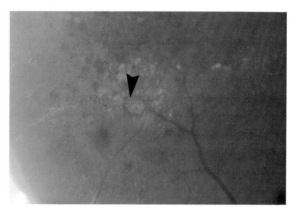

Figure 3.36   Typical "raspberry" lying in the area temporal to the macula (arrow)

they will again leak profusely into the retrovitreous space. The importance of the recognition of CNV is that they are extremely difficult to eliminate by regular photocoagulation and it is always necessary to perform direct photocoagulation of the CNV.

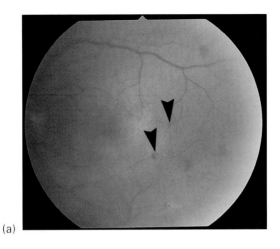

(a)

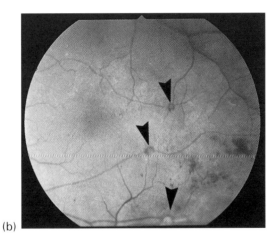

(b)

Figure 3.37 (a) Area temporal to the macula; it is difficult to identify the areas of "raspberry" formation; (b) red free photograph showing three raspberries (arrows); (c) fluorescein angiogram confirming the leaking "raspberries"

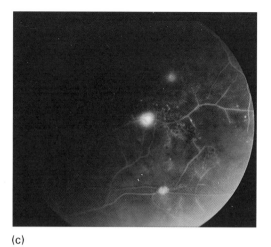

(c)

Figure 3.37   contd

New vessels on the disc

Flat NVD

In the presence of extensive peripheral capillary non-perfusion and when more than a quarter of the retina is non-perfused, NVD may develop. New vessels spreading from the disc and reaching out up to one disc diameter are also considered to be NVD and not NVE. NVD may be derived from the retinal or the choroidal circulation. To differentiate between these two sources of vessels, it is necessary to look at very early frames of the fluorescein angiogram.

The earliest vessels may be either in the centre of the disc or at the margin. Very fine early new vessels may be very difficult to distinguish from dilated capillaries, and it may be necessary to carry out fluorescein angiography to distinguish between the two (fig 3.38). On fluorescein angiography NVD will show staining and leakage whereas dilated capillaries will usually not leak, although they may stain minimally. NVD may sometimes be confused with the early development of collaterals; they tend to spread over the margin of the optic disc, whereas collaterals are confined to the disc surface itself

144

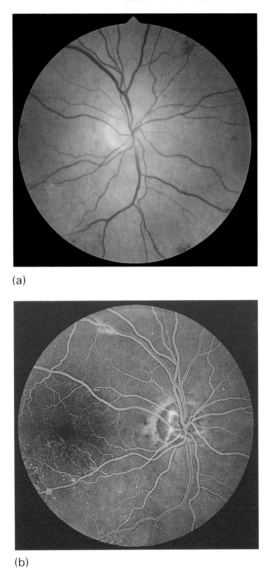

(a)

(b)

Figure 3.38   (a) Optic disc showing very fine vessels on the surface of the disc; (b) fluorescein angiogram of the optic disc confirms the leaking flat new vessels (fig 3.39). NVD from the optic disc spread slowly over the surface of the retina and have a predilection for extending along the major vascular arcades. The degree of leakage of disc vessels on fluorescein angiography is very variable; in some cases the leakage is minimal whereas in others there is profuse leakage. The degree of leakage corresponds to the maturity of the vessel and the degree of fibrous tissue around the vessel.

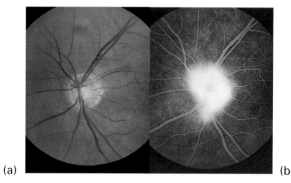

(a)   (b)

Figure 3.39   (a) Flat new vessels spreading over the surface of the optic disc; (b) fluorescein angiogram

Forward NVDs

NVD may extend forward from the surface of the retina along the stalk of detached posterior vitreous. Alternatively they may be pulled forward by the steady contraction of the vitreous or grow on the surface of the already detached vitreous. Once again, the vessels are most numerous in the area of the major vascular arcades, probably because of the greater attachment of vitreous to larger retinal vessels. On fluorescein angiography, forward NVD have a variable degree of fluorescence (fig 3.40). Those that are well established and mature tend to leak less than those that are newly formed.

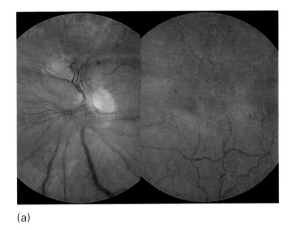

(a)

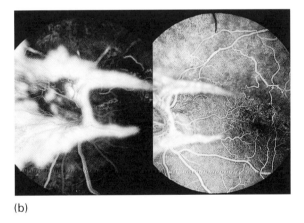

(b)

Figure 3.40 (a) New vessel attached to the posterior vitreous face, having been pulled forward from the optic disc; (b) fluorescein angiogram early in the later stage shows considerable leakage from these new vessels

Fibrous tissue

Fibrous tissue is a common accompaniment of either NVD or NVE (fig 3.41). Fibrous tissue may form at the site of any neovascular complex and may lie on the surface of the retina or extend forward to the posterior vitreous face. Fibrous tissue is more common on the vascular arcades where the

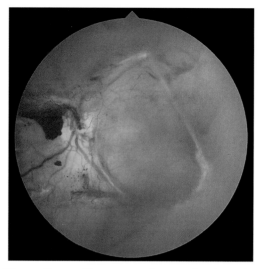

Figure 3.41 Fibrous tissue with new vessels extending from the optic disc. Contraction of the fibrous tissue has resulted in vitreous haemorrhage. Note that the fibrous tissue is beginning to form a ring around the posterior pole

where the vitreous is more firmly attached; ultimately it may extend as a complete ring around the posterior pole in the region of the temporal vascular arcades. Fibrous tissue contracts during its evolution and this may result in traction on new vessels pulling them off the surface of the retina; this may give rise to avulsion of vessels or to tractional retinal detachment with or without retinal hole formation. Similarly, during the course of contraction there may be disruption of new vessels, giving rise to haemorrhages into the retrovitreal space or into the vitreous gel.

The appearance of fibrosis is extremely variable. There may be diffuse or localised fibrosis. Clinically the changes may appear as bands running from the retina to the vitreous face, as is commonly seen in the stalk of new vessels coming off the optic disc. Fibrous tissue, as it forms on the posterior surface of the vitreous face, is almost always in the form of sheets which may be either diaphanous or opaque as a result of increased collagen content (figs 3.42–3.44). There may

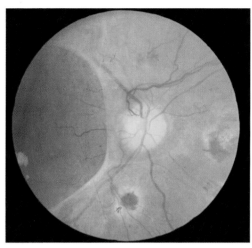

Figure 3.42 Large sheet of fibrous tissue extending across the posterior pole and extending around the upper and lower temporal vascular arcades

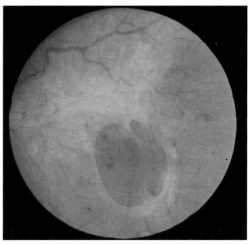

Figure 3.43 Large sheet of fibrous tissue extending across the posterior pole with condensation in various areas into bands

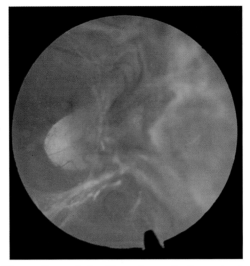

Figure 3.44   Fibrous tissue derived from the optic disc and extending to the nasal retina, causing a traction retinal detachment

also be more obvious thickenings in the sheet giving rise to the appearance that there are merely bands extending across the posterior vitreous face. These thickenings are always part of a more diffuse sheet.

With contraction of the fibrous tissue there may be detachment of the retina. The pattern of detachment may take on three different configurations:

1 A table top retinal detachment in which there is contraction of the fibrous tissue around the arcades resulting in detachment of the posterior pole. This results from multiple bands pulling at the vascular arcades or alternatively broad sheets on the major vessels.
2 Tangential traction: this tangential force on the retina results in a localised retinal detachment. This type of retinal detachment is frequently associated with hole formation giving rise to rhegmatogenous detachment. The distinction between traction without and that with hole formation is very distinct. In those in which no hole has formed the

surface of the retina, as viewed by the observer, tends to be either flat or concave whereas, if the hole has formed, then the retina has either a bullous or convex surface.

3 Anterior/posterior traction detachment: in this type of detachment the vitreous forces start at the vitreous base and extend posteriorly. If fibrous tissue involves the optic disc and extends towards the macula there may be distortion of macular anatomy giving rise to macular traction or, if the fibrous tissue is more extensive, the fovea itself may be detached and pulled towards the optic disc.

Preretinal traction membranes and macular pucker may occur following macular photocoagulation with attached vitreous. Fibrous tissue is not an indication for laser therapy. Active new vessels within the fibrous tissue should, however, be treated on their merits and the appropriate pattern of laser treatment performed. The question of the effect of laser therapy on contraction of fibrous tissue is debatable. In our experience fibrous tissue is relatively unaffected by small numbers of gentle photocoagulation burns. If many heavy burns are applied to the retina, however, we have seen extension and contraction of preretinal and forward fibrous tissue with the rapid progression to retinal detachment. Before photocoagulation it is often uncertain whether the fibrous tissue has undergone its entire evolution, and there may be further progression that is not related to laser therapy. If laser photocoagulation is required in patients with extensive fibrosis, it is best to apply laser treatment in several sessions. If perfused new blood vessels or haemorrhage is present in fibrous tissue and a blue–green or yellow laser is directed at these highly absorbing surfaces, this may result in contraction of the surrounding fibrosis. In some patients fibrous tissue may be present in the absence of any active neovascularisation but those patients may still go on to have occasional small vitreous haemorrhages. This is almost certainly the result of mechanical forces directed on either mature vessels within the fibrous tissue or the normal retinal vessels. In some patients with a detached vitreous gel, laser therapy may induce a contraction of the vitreous body. Although fibrous tissue accompanies new vessel development, this is frequently aggravated if there is accompanying vitreous haemorrhage or haemorrhages.

White vessels

A frequent accompaniment of vaso-occlusive disease in diabetic retinopathy is the presence of retinal white vessels (fig 3.45). These may be arteries, veins, or capillaries. The white vessel represents opacification of the vessel wall and the vessel is thinner than normal. These thin vessels are diagnostic of areas of capillary non-perfusion which can be demonstrated by fluorescein angiography. The vessel itself may be occluded, show perfusion, or absence of perfusion as a result of the lack of transparency of the vessel wall. White capillaries in the foveolar area will indicate non-perfusion and may confirm the cause of the visual loss

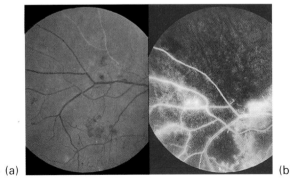

(a)   (b)

Figure 3.45 (a) White vessels extending superiorly in the supertemporal quadrant; (b) fluorescein angiogram shows complete capillary non-perfusion within this area

without the necessity for performing fluorescein angiography. Peripheral white vessels will be a marker for those non-perfusion areas that may require scatter treatment.

Retinal pigment epithelial appearance

A change in appearance of the RPE can occur in diabetic retinopathy. This change occurs in areas of capillary non-perfusion and is most commonly seen in the peripheral retina. In normal retina the appearance of the RPE is somewhat masked by the presence of the nerve fibre layer and ganglion cell layer. If these structures are absent, as may occur in areas of peripheral capillary non-perfusion, then the RPE is more readily seen and redder, and the pigment layer more obvious (fig 3.46). This change in the appearance of the RPE may be abrupt and in some patients a crenated edge can be seen at the junction of the normal and the abnormal retina. Accompanying this alteration in the RPE appearance there is a change in the larger blood vessels. In normal retina the margin of the red cell column is obscured by the presence of the superficial layers of the sensory retina. In the area in which this is absent there is no such attenuation and the vessel appears to stand out against the underlying pigment epithelium. The recognition of these subtle signs in the RPE colour and appearance of overlying blood vessels may be useful when giving scatter treatment to the peripheral retina because it is a marker of areas of capillary non-perfusion.

Posterior vitreous detachment

Posterior vitreous detachment in age or trauma related eyes tends to start in the upper periphery whereas in the diabetic

153

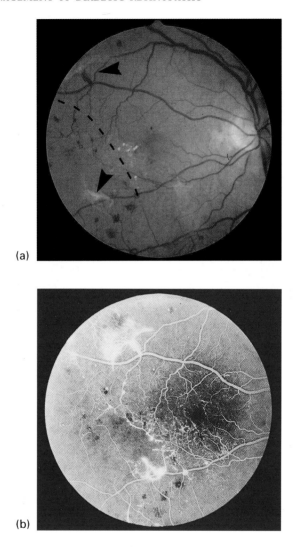

(a)

(b)

Figure 3.46 (a) Two small areas of preretinal new vessels (arrow). An area of altered colour appearance to the pigment epithelium: the greyer area is where the ganglion cell and nerve fibre layer are intact and the redder area, as indicated by the dashed line, shows an area where the pigment epithelium is no longer attenuated by the nerve fibre and ganglion cell layer. Also seen is a "raspberry" (arrow on (b)) confirmed on the accompanying fluorescein angiogram. (b) Fluorescein angiography confirms the presence of preretinal new vessels and shows the area of capillary non-perfusion at the site of the redder pigment epithelium

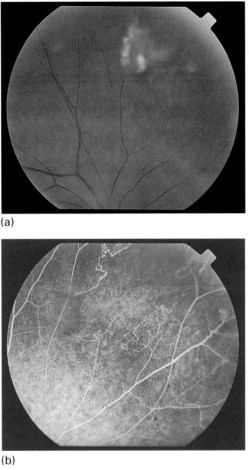

(a)

(b)

Figure 3.47 (a) Detached vitreous face, with a white area representing a previous preretinal new vessel. (b) The fluorescein angiogram shows the area of an avulsed vessel, not filling with fluorescein

eye it detaches in a more globular fashion, pulling away directly from the posterior pole. During detachment any structure that is attached, whether new vessels or fibrous tissue, will be pulled more forward than the surface of the retina. The pattern of changes thereafter depends on the degree and extent of this detachment. The vitreous body is more firmly attached to the retinal blood vessels, particularly the vessels of the temporal

155

arcades. Vitreous detachment can be induced by scatter photocoagulation. On rare occasions vitreous detachment may result in avulsion of the base of a new vessel complex from the retina, and this in turn will be seen as a ghost vessel lying across the posterior vitreous face (fig 3.47). If the vitreous has detached or partially detached and vitreous haemorrhages occur, then increased condensation of collagen may occur on the posterior vitreous face. If the vitreous is already detached, once new vessels begin to form, then the vessels will remain on the surface of the retina, and the ultimate prognosis is considerably improved.

4 Classification and treatment of diabetic retinopathy: diabetic maculopathy

Classification

The classification of diabetic retinopathy has evolved over the years with increasing knowledge of the pathological changes within the retina. The purpose of the classification is to develop guidelines as to the need for frequency of examination and follow up and also to define features that require particular forms or techniques of treatment. The most commonly used classification today is a modified Airlie House Classification as introduced by the ETDRS (Early Treatment Diabetic Retinopathy Study):

Non-proliferative diabetic retinopathy (NPDR)
Mild
Moderate
Severe
Proliferative diabetic retinopathy (PDR)
Early PDR
PDR with high risk criteria
PDR including advanced diabetic eye disease
Diabetic maculopathy
Macular oedema
Clinically significant macular oedema (CSMO)

Some of these stages are not mutually exclusive and may exist together, for example, moderate non-proliferative diabetic retinopathy and clinically significant macular oedema. The biomicroscopically visible changes of diabetic retinopathy are preceded by a stage of preretinopathy in which there are alterations within the flow and permeability of the retinal vessels. The preretinopathy leads on to the development of visible changes within the retina; these can be detected by ophthalmoscopic examination and also with fluorescein angiography. The development of diabetic retinopathy is a progressive event. The changes in the retinal capillary walls almost certainly develop gradually from the onset of diabetes mellitus and finally lead to capillary closure. Diabetic retinopathy is rare in type I diabetes mellitus before eight years of diabetic life; however, in type II diabetes mellitus, diabetic retinopathy may have been present for many years before diabetes was diagnosed, and therefore retinopathy could be present at the time of diagnosis or any time thereafter. The development of retinopathy is very variable in some patients; in 20% of patients diabetic retinopathy may be present after 10 years of diabetes, and in 80% after 20 years. After 30 years of diabetes mellitus almost all diabetic patients show at least some subtle signs of diabetic retinopathy.

Preretinopathy

One of the earliest reported features of preretinopathy has been the presence of dilated retinal veins. This is an extremely difficult sign to assess and its importance in clinical management is somewhat dubious. It has been shown that in the early preretinopathy stage there is increased retinal blood flow with decreased autoregulation in the retinal capillaries. It has, however, been well established that hyperglycaemia or even glucose transfusion may result in increased blood flow within the retinal circulation.

Vitreous fluorophotometry has been carried out in the preretinopathy stage of diabetic retinopathy and leakage of fluorescein has been shown to be one of the earliest changes that may occur before obvious microvascular lesions have developed. Fluorescein dye has been shown to leak from the retina into the vitreous, indicating an early breakdown in the blood–retina barrier.

Non-proliferative diabetic retinopathy

Mild non-proliferative diabetic retinopathy

Non-proliferative diabetic retinopathy (NPDR) may be of variable severity. The earliest visible changes that develop are microaneurysms, usually in the area temporal to the fovea representing mild NPDR, which does not require laser treatment. At this stage macular oedema with retinal thickening or hard exudate formation is rare but may be a threat to macular function, so there should be a follow up twice a year. If macular oedema becomes clinically significant, it should be lasered according to the guidelines given later in this book.

Moderate non-proliferative diabetic retinopathy

In addition to retinal microaneurysms, there may be other features elsewhere in the fundus, such as cotton wool spots, superficial flame shaped haemorrhages, or the more deeply placed blotch or cluster haemorrhages, venous dilatation, venous beading or loops, and intraretinal microvascular abnormalities (IRMA). If these changes are limited to two quadrants of the retina, this represents moderate NPDR. If these signs are present in more than two retinal quadrants, this represents severe NPDR.

If regular fluorescein angiography in patients with NPDR is carried out it is possible to identify lesions that will resolve and those that are developing. This is particularly true of retinal microaneurysms which tend to involute spontaneously as the result of thrombosis of either the microaneurysm or progression of capillary non-perfusion. In addition cotton wool spots may slowly resolve over a period of 3–6 months and they may show revascularisation or recanalisation.

Depending on the severity of the lesions that are present the follow up schedule is timed. If there are rapidly advancing areas of capillary non-perfusion, especially in type I diabetes, then follow up should be more frequent, that is, every three months. Such short term surveillance is also needed in type II diabetics with signs of moderate NPDR combined with diabetic macular oedema. As soon as macular oedema becomes clinically significant, it should be treated.

Severe non-proliferative diabetic retinopathy

Intraretinal microvascular abnormalities, venous beading, and severe amounts of blotch haemorrhages in more than two quadrants of the retina are a sign of retinal non-perfusion and ischaemia in the absence of neovascularisation, and hallmarks of severe NPDR. The clinical signs of retinal ischaemia can be variable but the severity tends to correlate with the overall area of capillary non-perfusion and speed of closure. Many of the signs of capillary non-perfusion can be subdivided into those indicating active or recent capillary closure, and chronic or long standing closure.

Clinical features of retinal ischaemia

Progressive closure
  IRMA
  Haemorrhages: cluster or blotch
  Venous abnormalities, beading
  Cotton wool spots
  Intracellular retinal oedema (cloudy swelling)

Chronic closure
  Venous abnormalities
    Beading
    Loops
  White vessels
  IRMA
  Change of RPE appearance

A mixture of active and chronic signs of retinal ischaemia may be present in the same eye or even in the same retinal quadrant. Where there is progressive and widespread ischaemia a fluorescein angiogram may be useful in delineating and confirming the extent of capillary non-perfusion, and could reveal tiny new vessels that had been missed on clinical examination. Where there is clinical doubt an angiogram will also help to distinguish IRMA from preretinal new vessels. In IRMA a spidery network of vessels is typically seen in the early frames of the transit and, if present, leakage is limited to the growing tips. Preretinal new vessels, conversely, show early and progressive leakage of fluorescein from the initial branching trunk to the most distal terminals. Again, clinically significant macular oedema (CSMO), if present, requires appropriate focal or grid therapy.

Management of severe NPDR

The ETDRS results suggest that panretinal photo-coagulation may be considered in patients with severe NPDR, although they are somewhat inconclusive in this respect. A number of factors need, however, to be considered in planning the appropriate management for such a patient. Associated risk factors such as type I diabetes mellitus, arterial hypertension, pregnancy, lack of compliance, and diabetic nephropathy could not only lead to a decision leaning towards panretinal mild scatter photocoagulation, but also determine the frequency of follow up examinations. The status of the fellow eye and eye at risk needs to be evaluated carefully. Finally, severe NPDR needs to be assessed—whether there is progressive or long standing capillary closure. Not all patients with severe NPDR share the same natural history and three subgroups are of interest:

1 Type I diabetic patients with severe NPDR
2 Type I diabetic patients with CSMO and severe NPDR
3 Type II diabetic patients with CSMO and severe NPDR.

Type I diabetes with severe NPDR   Severe NPDR may be particularly progressive in patients with type I diabetes and early recognition is essential for effective management. At presentation both retinas usually appear similarly affected, with multiple areas of deep blotch haemorrhages, although interspersed IRMA and cotton wool spots are also common. Parts of the midperipheral retina may be oedematous. Fluorescein angiography reveals a characteristic pattern of peripheral capillary non-perfusion. In the majority, the arterioles and venules remain patent within the areas of non-perfusion. These small patent vessels tend to be dilated and stain; they leak during the latter stages of the angiogram, giving the appearance of smudged vessel walls. Leaking microaneurysms are seen around the areas of non-perfusion. This kind of severe NPDR is rapidly progressive and neovascularisation inevitably develops, usually within a few months. Furthermore once proliferative retinopathy is established, subsequent control with panretinal photocoagulation is often difficult. As a result of this, in these cases we would advocate mild scatter panretinal photocoagulation before the onset of neovascularisation. Treatment should be applied specifically to the widespread areas of capillary non-perfusion in the midperipheral and peripheral retina, starting on the nasal side.

By contrast another group of type I diabetic patients shares similar features of retinal ischaemia, although the progression of the retinopathy is more heterogeneous. The progression rate of capillary closure is slow and intermittent. Some eyes do eventually develop NVE, but most never progress to high risk PDR.

The clinical signs in this group usually demonstrate a mixture of recent and long standing signs of ischaemia. Furthermore the lesions may demonstrate different stages of evolution, for example, some cotton wool spots are clearing as others appear. Again IRMA and venous abnormalities, such as beading and loops, are typical. The appearance of increased numbers of blotch haemorrhages usually signifies progression of the retinopathy with an increased risk of neovascularisation. On fluorescein angiography the areas of capillary non-perfusion are initially small and discrete. In progressive disease areas of non-perfusion develop and extend with adjacent areas coalescing to involve progressively larger areas of the retina. As capillary closure becomes more widespread obliteration of the smaller arterioles and venules occurs. Although this is often best seen on fluorescein angiography, closure of the smaller vessels may be clinically recognised as "white lines."

Management of this type of severe NPDR is controversial. Early, mild, scatter, panretinal photocoagulation may prevent or delay the development of neovascularisation, although the preferred option is regular clinical review and withholding laser treatment until the development of new vessels. This approach is probably best unless there is evidence of rapid and progressive capillary closure in a patient who is a poor attender. If mild, scatter, panretinal treatment is undertaken, the laser can be directed to the areas of capillary non-perfusion as a so called "modified" panretinal photo-coagulation.

Type I diabetes with CSMO and severe NPDR CSMO with focal leakage from microaneurysms and circinate rings in young diabetic subjects is relatively uncommon, but when present is often associated with widespread peripheral capillary closure. Generally this group of patients presents with symptoms of blurred vision and small central microscotomata. In most cases the symptoms are not severe and may only produce minor difficulties for reading or other near vision tasks.

The threat to vision for these patients is not only from the macular oedema but also from accelerating capillary closure. The signs of capillary closure in this group are usually more subtle. The appearance of large tracts of non-perfused capillary crisscrossed by patent arterioles and venules is, however, characteristic of this group. The larger vessels stain with fluorescein as they cross the non-perfused areas, giving the vessel walls a smudgy appearance.

The association of impending NVD or NVE and macular oedema in the young diabetic subject has a poor prognosis (fig 4.1). The new vessels are often rapidly progressive and resistant to panretinal laser treatment. Mild scatter panretinal photocoagulation before the onset of neovascularisation does appear to protect this group and often prevents the otherwise inevitable progression from severe non-proliferative to proliferative retinopathy. If there is focal CSMO, treatment of this should be delayed until the effect of the PRP has become established. In most eyes the CSMO will resolve spontaneously without the need for any focal laser treatment.

Type II diabetes with CSMO and severe NPDR In adult onset diabetes, macular oedema is the pre-eminent vision threatening retinal change. Capillary non-perfusion may, however, develop or coexist in these eyes and progress to proliferative retinopathy. In most of these patients peripheral closure is very slow to develop and the features characteristic of this kind of diabetic retinopathy indicate that there has been chronic retinal hypoperfusion. If neovascularisation develops in this group it is not particularly aggressive. Fluorescein angiography reveals a different pattern of non-perfusion from that seen in the younger group. In these older patients there is, in addition to capillary non-perfusion, closure of the arterioles and venules; unlike some of the other groups, the tracts of capillary non-perfusion are not crisscrossed with patent vessels.

Prophylactic panretinal photocoagulation for patients who have adult onset diabetes with macular oedema and severe NPDR is generally not advocated for two reasons:

1 These patients are already under short term surveillance for their macular oedema, facilitating the early diagnosis of proliferative retinopathy.
2 As macular function is already compromised, prophylactic panretinal photocoagulation may further restrict visual function as a result of further breakdown of the blood–retina barrier, thus increasing macular oedema.

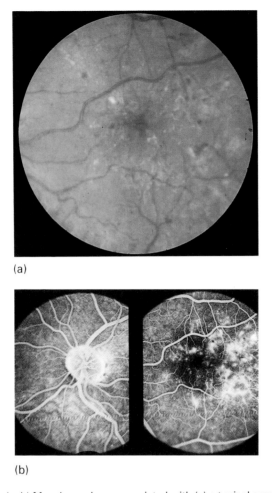

(a)

(b)

Figure 4.1 (a, b) Macular oedema associated with (c) a typical smudgy type of peripheral capillary non-perfusion with aneurysms. (d, e) Following 2500 panretinal photocoagulation burns; in spite of this new vessels developed on the optic disc and subsequently needed a further 3500 laser burns to control these new vessels. (f, g) The focal macular oedema was treated by additional focal laser treatment to the site of leakage

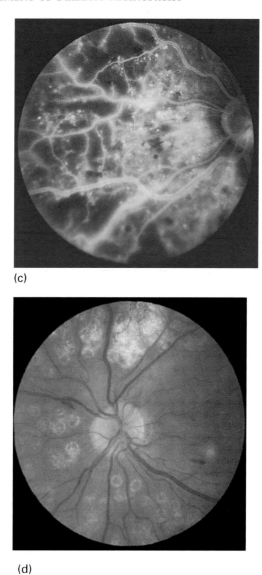

(c)

(d)

Figure 4.1   contd

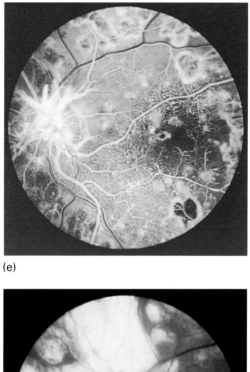

(e)

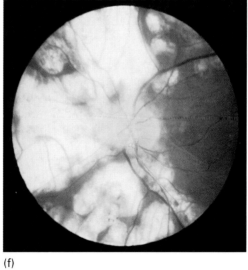

(f)

Figure 4.1   contd

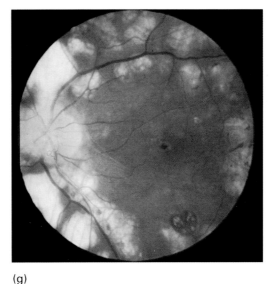

(g)

Figure 4.1 contd

If the macular oedema appears, however, as clinically significant it has to be treated instantly, and panretinal treatment should be delayed until neovascularisation develops.

Diabetic macular oedema

Diabetic macular oedema is defined as hard exudate and retinal thickening involving the macular area. Although these features lie in the macular area the fovea is not yet involved.

The oedema could be derived from leakage from the retinal vessels and/or through the RPE (deep leakage). On top of this, visual loss may be worsened by capillary closure involving the foveal capillary arcade—so called ischaemic maculopathy.

Treatment should be considered in those eyes in which there is visual loss as a consequence of macular oedema or in those eyes in which there is clinically significant macular oedema, which is defined as retinal thickening or hard exudate formation within 500 μm of the centre of the fovea (fig 4.2). Patients with macular oedema most commonly have had non-insulin dependent adult onset diabetes mellitus, or presumed diabetes, for over eight years. Macular oedema may also occur in those patients with insulin dependent, juvenile onset diabetes, although this is sometimes a manifestation of associated peripheral capillary closure. In this group the macular changes may precede the onset of neovascularisation. The factors initiating macular oedema include duration of diabetes, poor diabetic control, arterial hypertension, hyperlipidaemia, and diabetic nephropathy. Patients with macular problems may be divided into four subgroups, each group having different features, course of disease, and requirement for laser treatment. The clinical features in the subtypes of diabetic maculopathy reflect the underlying pathological processes which can be purely leakage, or ischaemia, but may be a varying combination. Sometimes the pattern of maculopathy is not apparent without the use of fluorescein angiography.

Classification of diabetic maculopathy and macular oedema

- Focal exudative macular oedema
- Diffuse exudative macular oedema
- Ischaemic maculopathy
- Mixed forms

Focal exudative diabetic macular oedema

This group of patients with macular oedema has the characteristic features of well defined focal areas of leakage with retinal thickening; these areas are often surrounded by circinate hard exudates. In focal exudative macular oedema, discrete leakage sites are a consistent feature. Leakage may occur from retinal microaneurysms or areas of dilated retinal capillaries. The extent of the vascular changes is very variable, with anything from as few as one or two retinal micro-aneurysms with minimal retinal thickening to associated widespread haemorrhage and intraretinal hard exudate formation. Leakage from capillaries can occur from the deep or superficial capillary network in the retina. Leakage from either microvascular abnormality gives rise to intraretinal oedema with a bulk fluid flow towards competent capillaries. At these distal sites the fluid in the extracellular space is reabsorbed into the relatively normal retinal capillary bed, causing the deposition and accumulation of the large molecules such as proteins and lipids—seen as hard exudates.

The exact configuration of the exudate depends not only on the degree and sites of leakage, but also on the characteristics of fluid movement and absorption. Accordingly hard exudates found at the macula vary considerably. In some areas small (10 µm) microdots are seen representing macrophages full of lipoprotein. In other eyes the hard exudate at the fovea may have a linear distribution, irregularly arranged or in an annular pattern (fig 4.4 (b)). The turnover of intraretinal hard exudate is slow and is measured in months or years. In situations where there is continued leakage an equilibrium is reached and the hard exudate no longer increases in size.

In many patients with focal exudative macular oedema the areas of leakage are well away from the fovea, and central vision may be preserved. This is when macular oedema is not clinically significant. Most patients in this group are asymptomatic, although some may complain of fluctuations in visual acuity or paracentral scotomata. In those patients with disturbed central vision, the degree of visual loss is usually related to the extent of retinal oedema and hard exudate formation. Once retinal thickening or hard exudates are coming as close as 500 µm to the centre of the fovea (CSMO), focal laser treatment must be performed, even in patients with perfect vision (figs 4.2 and 4.3).

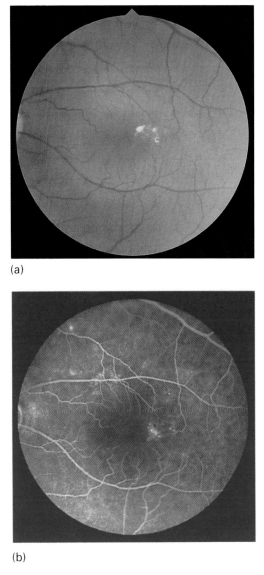

(a)

(b)

Figure 4.2 (a) Retina before treatment for paramacular microaneurysms associated with CSMO; (b) fluorescein angiogram. (c, d) Six months after treating, showing resolution of oedema and exudates

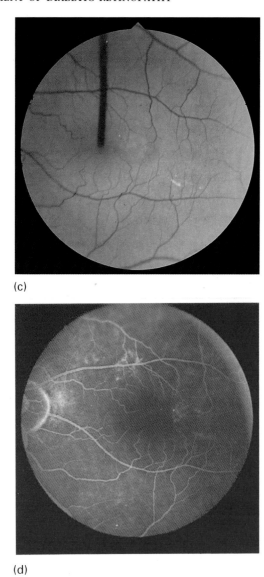

(c)

(d)

Figure 4.2 contd

Direct focal treatment to leaking microaneurysms
(table 4.1) The aim of treatment is to stop the leakage from the microvascular abnormalities and to allow hard exudates and fluid to be absorbed. Patients with focal exudative diabetic macular oedema require treatment if areas of hard exudate or retinal thickening encroach within 500 μm of the fovea (CSMO), with or without visual loss. Treatment should be applied to leaking microvascular lesions and to achieve this goal it is often useful to have a fluorescein angiogram available at the time of treatment. An angiogram is particularly useful when it is suspected that these leaking lesions themselves are very close to the fovea.

Table 4.1   Treatment parameters for direct focal photocoagulation

Spot size	50–100 μm
Exposure time	0·1 s
Power	Just for minimal blanching of the RPE or blanching of the microaneurysm
Wavelength	To blanch the RPE: 514 nm, 532 nm, 577 nm, 647 nm, 810 nm To blanch microaneurysms: 514 nm, 532 nm, 577 nm

Laser may be applied to those leaking sites that are close enough to the central capillary arcade to contribute to the macular oedema. In treating any source of leakage the power of the laser should be just sufficient to produce a minimal reaction.

Long wavelength light (red or infrared) has the theoretical advantage of reduced absorption by the xanthophyll pigment. In practice the dye laser tuned to 514 or 577 nm provides a satisfactory burn at low powers. The argon green, the doubled frequency Nd:YAG with 532 nm, and the 577 nm dye laser are the lasers of choice if blanching of the retinal micro-aneurysm is regarded as the ideal end point.

There are, however, two complementary techniques for photocoagulation in patients with focal exudative macular oedema: direct blanching of the vascular lesion or treatment of the RPE underneath. To treat retinal microaneurysms

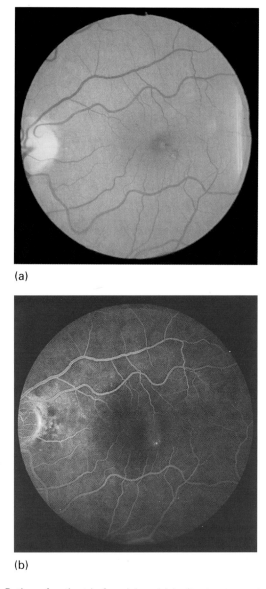

(a)

(b)

Figure 4.3   Retina of patient before (a) and (c) after treatment in a patient with a small area of microaneurysms immediately adjacent to the fovea. (b, d) Fluorescein angiograms before and after respectively. This treatment resulted in resolution of the oedema and improvement in visual acuity

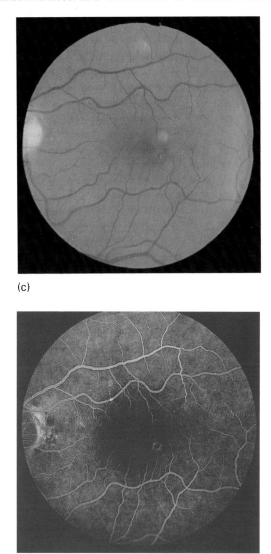

(c)

(d)

Figure 4.3   contd

directly, a small spot size (50 or 100 µm) is used. The intensity of the reaction should be sufficient to produce a visible change in the microaneurysm. The microaneurysm will either darken or blanch. Occasionally, after treatment a pale halo will surround the microaneurysm. It is important with this technique to focus the laser carefully on the retinal microaneurysm and so minimise any "splash" on the adjacent RPE. As a consequence of the higher laser energies required to blanch the microaneurysm, unintended horizontal spread of energy could occur, damaging the neighbouring sensory retina.

More recent studies have shown that blanching of the microaneurysm itself, through the use of a laser wavelength that is directly absorbed within haemoglobin, is not mandatory to cause subsequent closure of the retinal vascular lesions. Alternatively, mild treatment of the RPE underlying a retinal microaneurysm, using just a single burn with the near infrared diode laser at 810 nm, also causes angiographically proven regression of the retinal microaneurysm and stops the leakage within weeks. This is a very gentle mode of treatment which causes less damage to the sensory retina, and it is extremely helpful when treating in close proximity to the fovea. The mechanism of action of this new technique is not as yet completely understood. There is a hypothesis that there are vasoinhibitory factors released from the RPE which mediate closure of the retinal microaneurysms.

Indirect focal treatment (table 4.2)   For treating larger areas of leakage, that is, the inner field of large circinate rings, with multiple leaking sites, a larger spot size, such as 200 µm, is best to perform a grid type treatment within a large area of focal leakage. In these cases the laser is focused on the RPE beneath the leaking area. Again the intensity of the laser should be just sufficient to produce moderate blanching of the RPE. The exact amount of energy required will depend on the degree of oedema and the extent of scatter by the semiopaque intraretinal fluid. With this technique the burn can indirectly coagulate the source of leakage or induce closure of the overlying vasculature by releasing vaso-inhibitory growth factors from the RPE, depending on the power employed. This method of treatment is best reserved for large circinate rings (fig 4.4).

Table 4.2   Treatment parameters for indirect focal photocoagulation

Spot size	200 μm
Exposure time	0·1 s
Power	Just for minimal blanching of the RPE
Wavelength	All available wavelengths except argon (488 nm)

In many eyes a combination of direct and indirect focal treatment patterns is used, the small spot size focal treatment being used in areas close to the fovea and the larger spot size outside this area. The response to treatment in this group of patients depends on the degree of foveolar involvement. The best results are obtained in those eyes with well defined, circinate, hard exudate rings, but minor or no involvement of the fovea and good vision. The poorest response is seen in eyes in which central vision is reduced as a result of a foveal plaque of hard exudate or massive long standing cystoid oedema; although this may reabsorb following laser treatment, the vision will remain poor (fig 4.5).

In essence, it is easier to preserve good visual acuity than to regain visual acuity that has been previously lost. Thus, treatment should be performed when retinal thickening and hard exudate approach the fovea, but when the foveola is not yet thickened. Once the foveola is involved and long standing cystoid macular oedema has formed, the prognosis is poor.

Patients should be re-evaluated one month after treatment. Any residual oedma should be assessed and any additional leaking points should be considered for treatment. It is not uncommon for more retinal microaneurysms to be seen at this visit, because they will have become visible as the surrounding semiopaque oedema subsides. An increase in

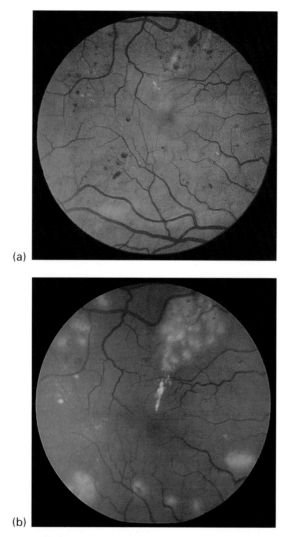

Figure 4.4 (a) Moderate non-proliferative diabetic retinopathy without any clinically significant oedema and normal vision. (b) Six months later the exudates had now spread to within 500 μm of the fovea, with associated clinically significant macular oedema, and the laser burns arrowed can be seen applied to the areas of microvascular leakage. (c) Three months later the exudates are slowly resolving and (d) six months later the exudates have completely resolved and all that remains is the photocoagulation scar.

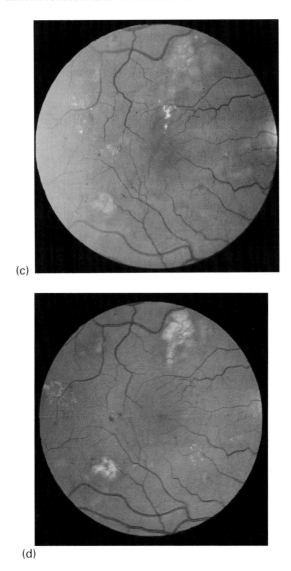

(c)

(d)

Figure 4.4 contd

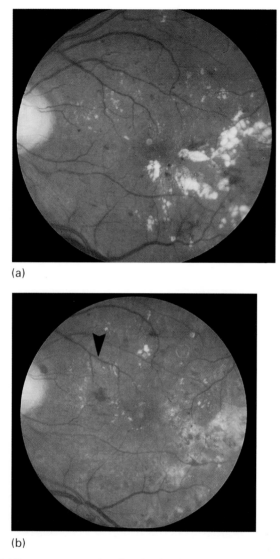

(a)

(b)

Figure 4.5 (a) Pre-treatment retina showing hard exudates and, in addition, retinal microaneurysms very close to the fovea. The technique employed was both the direct and the indirect treatment with the direct method to the lesions close to the fovea, and the indirect method to the lesions temporal to the fovea. (b) Appearance some six months after the initial treatment, and note (arrow) a further area of leakage on the papillar–macular bundle. (c, d) The macular oedema has gradually resolved

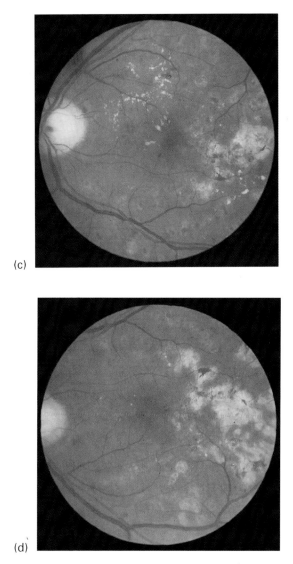

(c)

(d)

Figure 4.5 contd

hard exudate may also be seen, reflecting reabsorption of retinal oedema with consequent lipoprotein precipitation. This observation has implications for those patients with hard exudate lying close to the fovea before laser treatment.

181

Under such conditions we recommend fractionation of the treatment—delivering the total treatment over some weeks. Follow up visits should be scheduled at three week intervals, depending on the severity of macular oedema and the primary response to treatment. Any persistence or additional area of leakage must be treated if there is a threat to central vision. Fluorescein angiography may again be of use in some cases, although interpretation of the angiogram is often difficult as a result of hyperfluorescence associated with the previous laser burns. If fluorescein angiography is to be performed it is necessary to ensure that early pictures are taken before there is significant hyperfluorescence in the RPE adjacent to the previous burns. Stereo pictures will also assist in determining the site of leakage.

Diffuse diabetic macular oedema

In some diabetic patients leakage occurs diffusely from the retinal capillaries. In these patients retinal microaneurysms tend to be few in number, although there may be a combination of retinal microaneurysms in one area and leaking capillaries in another. Similarly hard exudate and intraretinal haemorrhages tend to be few in number and small in size.

Often the patient presenting with diffuse macular oedema will admit to only a recent but rapid loss of visual acuity although on examination the visual acuity is rarely better than 6/18. It is difficult to explain this feature but it may represent a sudden decompensation of the retinal capillaries. Patients with diffuse macular oedema almost always have maturity onset diabetes and often have coexistent arterial hypertension.

The extent of oedema in patients with diffuse macular oedema is variable; it may occupy much of the posterior pole or a smaller region of the macula. In most cases cystoid macular oedema is the main feature, together with a small amount of haemorrhage. On occasions there is haemorrhage into the cystoid spaces. Hard exudate is not characteristic, although it can be seen at the junction of normal and abnormal retinal capillaries.

Patients with diffuse macular oedema can be subdivided according to the site and degree of leakage. The purpose of this classification is to provide a rationale for appropriate treatment.

- Central diffuse
- Generalised diffuse

Central diffuse diabetic macular oedema This subdivision is characterised by leakage of the capillaries immediately adjacent to the foveal arcade. The degree of oedema is variable, but remains localised to the fovea. Cystoid oedema is frequently seen. Fluorescein angiography of this group of patients typically shows leakage from the dilated capillaries surrounding the fovea. The fluorescein dye may accumulate in the petaloid pattern of cystoid macular oedema (fig 4.6).

Generalised diffuse diabetic macular oedema Generalised diffuse macular oedema is characterised by widespread retinal thickening across the entire posterior pole, extending far beyond the fovea. This type of diffuse oedema tends to be bilateral. In these patients the visual acuity is worse than 6/18. Retinal microaneurysms, intraretinal haemorrhages, and hard exudates tend to be less frequent in this group, perhaps reflecting greater obscuration by the semiopaque fluid.

Fluorescein angiography may reveal more retinal microaneurysms than were clinically apparent, but again the overriding feature is capillary dilatation and subsequent profuse leakage. On occasions it is possible to identify hyperfluorescence, seen only during the early stages of the angiogram, at the level of the RPE, suggesting that at least some of the oedema is derived from the choroid (fig 4.9).

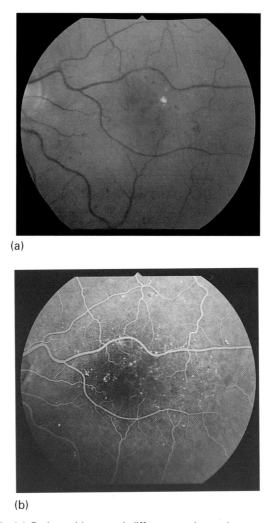

(a)

(b)

Figure 4.6 (a) Retina with central diffuse macular oedema pre-treatment showing leakage from capillaries immediately surrounding the fovea with (b) accompanying fluorescein angiogram; (c, d) early and (e, f) late response to laser treatment with drying up of the macula

The leakage of fluid from the capillaries in this type of oedema shares many of the features of macular oedema seen in other maculopathies, such as macular oedema following central retinal vein occlusion, retinal telangiectasia, and

184

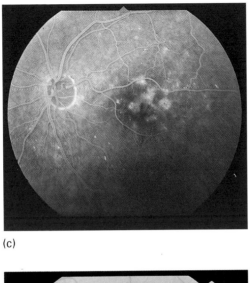

(c)

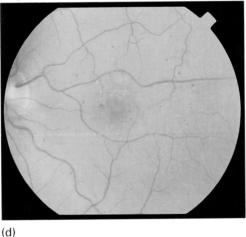

(d)

Figure 4.6   contd

aphakic cystoid macular oedema, and such secondary causes
of macular oedema should be ruled out before treatment is
initiated. In addition diffuse oedema may occur following
panretinal photocoagulation, particularly in those who have
been re-treated. Occasionally, diffuse macular oedema may

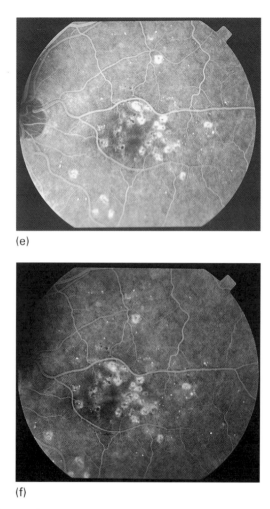

(e)

(f)

Figure 4.6 contd

be mimicked by ischaemic diabetic maculopathy. Closure of the parafoveolar capillaries may lead to swelling of the ganglion cell and nerve fibre layer and could be clinically indistinguishable from diffuse oedema. As a result of the difficulty in establishing the diagnosis of generalised diffuse

186

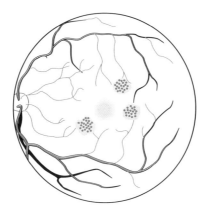

Figure 4.7 Diagrammatic representation of the method of treatment for focal diabetic maculopathy. Laser burns (green) are applied to the leaking focuses, leaving 500 µm between burns

macular oedema we recommend that a full medical history and examination should be taken, and advocate the use of fluorescein angiography in all cases.

Treatment for diffuse diabetic macular oedema

Photocoagulation for diffuse macular oedema has been empirically derived, but a number of controlled trials have shown a "grid pattern" of lasering to be effective in the control of the diffuse type of oedema. In essence, the laser is applied to the oedematous area in the posterior pole using a 100–200 µm spot size, taking care to avoid the foveal and parafoveal areas (fig 4.10). A burn with a short exposure and a low intensity is recommended—just sufficient to cause a threshold burn at the level of the RPE. The power setting will depend on the quantity and opaqueness of the oedematous fluid, the laser wavelength employed, and the degree of scatter by the fluid. The exact configuration of the grid depends on the pattern of leakage. In patients with diffuse generalised macular oedema, 100–200 burns will be required, spaced by intervals of a size corresponding to the diameter of the spot (fig 4.11).

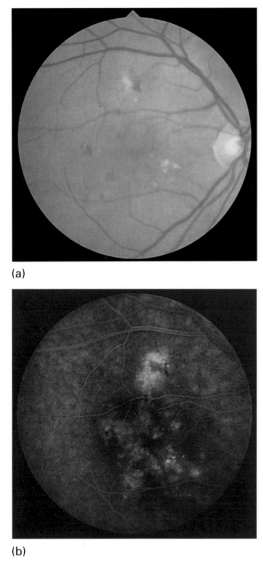

(a)

(b)

Figure 4.8 (a) In this patient there are areas of central leakage surrounding the posterior pole with virtually no evidence of any exudate formation, in spite of quite marked leakage on the fluorescein angiogram (b). (c, d) Appearance post-treatment with drying up of the retina, and maintenance of visual acuity

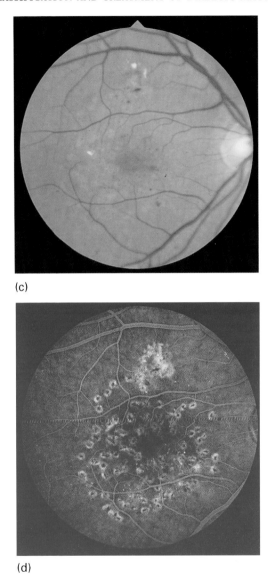

(c)

(d)

Figure 4.8   contd

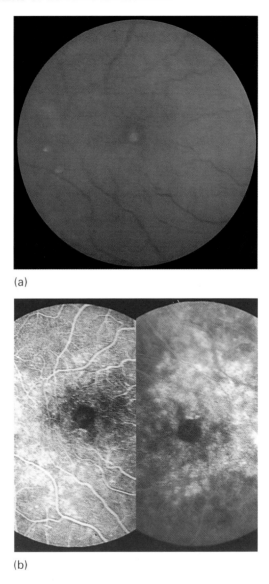

(a)

(b)

Figure 4.9 (a) Diffuse generalised macular oedema; (b) fluorescein angiogram showing extensive capillary dilatation and leakage, and in the early stages of the angiogram a possible leakage through the pigment epithelium

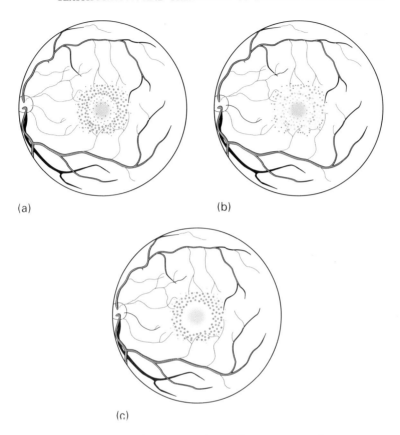

(a)

(b)

(c)

Figure 4.10 Diagrammatic representation of the treatment and re-treatment for generalised diffuse macular oedema. (a) Grid treatment pattern; (b) scarring of the grid laser burns, but residual cystoid macular oederna in the centre; (c) additional laser burns close to the foveal avascular arcade

It is best to apply the full grid therapy in one sitting, but only one eye at a time. The response to treatment can be assessed after one month by comparing the retinal thickening. If the oedema persists re-treatment in a similar fashion is indicated. On occasion, the diffuse macular oedema resolves but visual acuity remains unchanged. This reflects irreversible damage to the photoreceptors, although the integrity of the blood–retina barrier has been re-established.

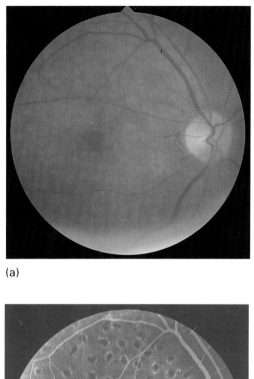

(a)

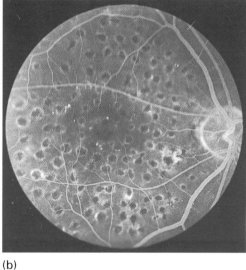

(b)

Figure 4.11   (a) Grid laser treatment and (b) fluorescein angiogram; (c) some six months later the grid has become much more obvious

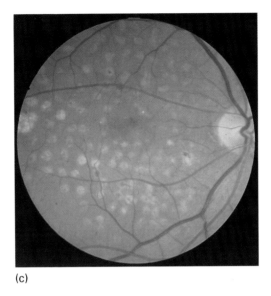

(c)

Figure 4.11   contd

Treatment to the fellow eye should be considered after one eye has been fully treated. This policy minimises patient dissatisfaction and encourages the patient to take an active role in the decision making process. If the patient is able to visualise the grid pattern of scotomata, as sometimes seen after this mode of treatment, he or she may elect not to have treatment to the fellow eye. Furthermore, subretinal neovascularisation and preretinal traction membranes may develop as a complication of treatment and, together with failure of a functional improvement, this may signify a poor prognosis for the fellow eye.

The response to grid treatment is very variable. In some eyes there is significant improvement in vision, whereas in others the vision remains unchanged. In some cases the grid will produce a satisfactory response in the area treated, but leave a central oedematous area with cystoid foveal oedema (see fig 4.10). In these patients it may be useful to extend the laser grid almost up to the central capillary arcade.

Grid laser photocoagulation works independently of the laser wavelength employed (table 4.3).

Table 4.3 Treatment parameters for grid photocoagulation

Spot size	100–200 μm
Exposure time	0·05–0·1 s
Power	Just for minimal blanching of the RPE
Dye	All available wavelengths except argon (488 nm)

Ischaemic diabetic maculopathy

This can be divided into central and peripheral patterns. In patients with ischaemic diabetic maculopathy the predominant clinical finding is macular capillary non-perfusion. This type of diabetic maculopathy occurs predominantly in the non-insulin dependent patient. The accompanying oedema may be variable, reflecting the degree of incompetence of the residual capillaries. If there are no capillaries left at the fovea, and the outer blood–retinal barrier is intact, the fovea may be dry.

With careful observation the features of capillary non-perfusion can be seen by stereoscopic biomicroscopy. Small white vessels may be seen radiating around the fovea and deep blotch haemorrhages are not uncommon. Cotton wool spots between the temporal arcades reflect ischaemia, although this may not extend to involve the fovea. Similarly NVD or NVE may alert the examiner to widespread peripheral areas of ischaemia which could involve the fovea.

Central ischaemic diabetic maculopathy Ischaemic diabetic maculopathy can be subdivided into a central group where the ischaemia starts at the fovea and spreads in a centrifugal manner, involving progressively greater areas of the retina. In this group of patients there is early visual loss, although this is usually not severe. Often retinal microaneurysms are seen at the peripheral extent of the closure (fig 4.12).

Peripheral ischaemic diabetic maculopathy In the second group there is peripheral capillary non-perfusion which extends to the posterior pole. Often the ischaemia is more irregular around the fovea with the area temporal to the fovea being preferentially involved. In this group the visual acuity tends to be poor and there is a greater risk of either NVD or NVE (fig 4.13).

As a result of the difficulty in clinically assessing ischaemic maculopathy most patients require fluorescein angiography to define the pattern and extent of non-perfusion. Patients with large areas of non-perfusion should be closely reviewed for neovascularisation.

Treatment of ischaemic diabetic maculopathy Many treatment approaches have been advocated for patients with ischaemic diabetic maculopathy. Grid treatment and horse-shoe patterns of photocoagulation have been tried without any success. Panretinal photocoagulation has been advocated as a means of diverting retinal blood flow to the posterior pole, but this has also been abandoned as it has been shown to cause increased leakage from the capillaries around the fovea. Panretinal photocoagulation is, however, required when neovascularisation coexists.

We have not, however, found any treatment pattern that is useful in patients with solitary central or peripheral ischaemic diabetic maculopathy. Although eyes with peripheral capillary closure have a greater risk of developing neovascularisation than the central group, we do not advocate prophylactic panretinal photocoagulation. Panretinal treatment should be considered for only those patients who have already developed new vessels or subsequently develop new vessels.

Mixed diabetic maculopathy

Many patients with maculopathy have features of more than one type of maculopathy. There is usually a variable degree of hard exudate, retinal thickening, retinal

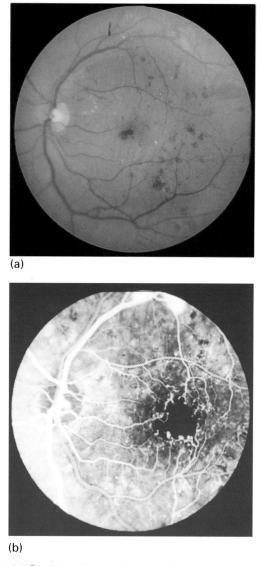

(a)

(b)

Figure 4.12   (a) Exudates, haemorrhages, and microaneurysms; (b) fluorescein angiogram shows widespread capillary closure temporal to the fovea; some widening of the central foveal avascular zone (FAZ), a small "raspberry" in the area immediately at the upper vascular arcade, and widespread peripheral capillary closure

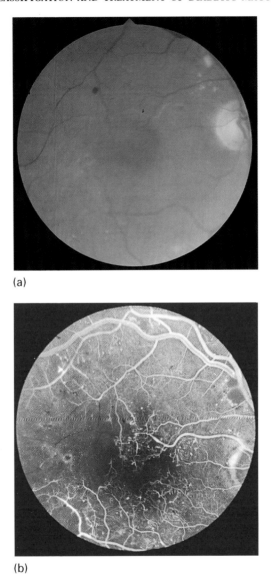

(a)

(b)

Figure 4.13 (a) Relatively featureless fundus, although note the white vessel going across the macula. (b) Fluorescein angiogram showing extensive closure in the periphery temporal to the fovea and contiguous with the closure in the central area

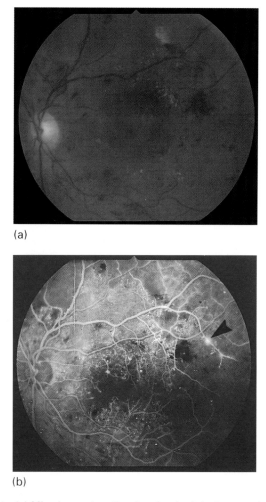

(a)

(b)

Figure 4.14 (a) Mixed maculopathy showing both leakage and closure. (b) The fluorescein angiogram confirms this and also shows a small "raspberry" (arrow) developing in the area temporal to the macula

microaneurysms, and retinal haemorrhages of the deeper cluster, superficial, or even diffuse type. Cotton wool spots may also be present. The visual acuity is generally poor. On fluorescein angiography the appearance is often variable with multifocal leakage, some diffuse areas of leakage often being

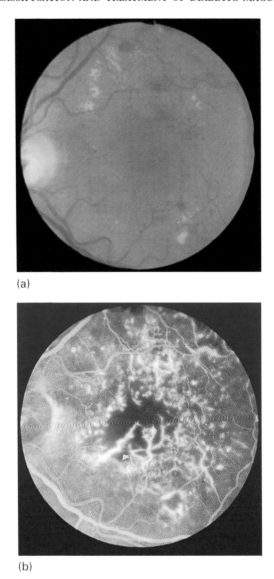

(a)

(b)

Figure 4.15 (a) Mixed maculopathy with exudates and CSMO; (b, c) fluorescein angiogram shows closure, widening of the FAZ, and late leakage both above and below the macula. (d) After grid laser treatment applied directly to the area of leakage; (e, f) early and late fluorescein angiograms showing the almost complete resolution of the leakage

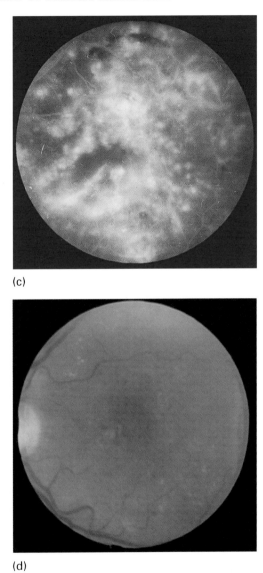

(c)

(d)

Figure 4.15   contd

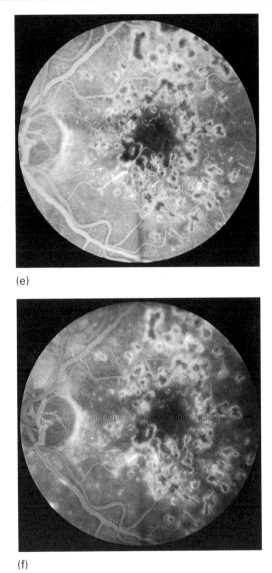

(e)

(f)

Figure 4.15   contd

interspersed with areas of capillary non-perfusion (fig 4.14). Fluorescein angiography is, however, essential for an accurate assessment before treatment. The early frames are most important for interpretation, because later, in the transit of dye, leakage may obscure microvascular detail. In most, as a result of widening of the foveal capillary arcade or extensive cystoid macular oedema, laser treatment is unlikely to be of any value. This is especially true if the fovea has a plaque of hard exudate or a pigmented scar. Some patients may, however, benefit from focal treatment to the leaking areas, hopefully to reduce the amount of macular oedema. Again this group may also have coexistent peripheral capillary non-perfusion and it is important to exclude neovascularisation which will require panretinal treatment on its own merits.

Treatment of mixed diabetic maculopathy   The treatment technique in this group depends on the site and extent of leakage. If leaking retinal microaneurysms are present, then they should receive focal treatment; if there are areas of diffuse capillary leakage then these areas should receive grid treatment. The decision to treat in this group is often difficult to make, but on occasion it is possible to effect some drying of the retina with maintenance of visual acuity (fig 4.15).

5 Classification and treatment of diabetic retinopathy: proliferative diabetic retinopathy

Classification

Proliferative diabetic retinopathy
New vessels elsewhere (NVE)
New disc vessels (NVD)

High risk proliferative diabetic retinopathy
New vessels (NVE/NVD)
Preretinal haemorrhage

In diabetic retinopathy progressive occlusion of the retinal microcirculation can lead to a number of clinical patterns of retinopathy. Recognition of these patterns is important, not only for planning management, but because it often enables an accurate prognosis to be given to the patient.

In diabetic patients retinal ischaemia is present in severe non-proliferative (NPDR) and proliferative diabetic retinopathy (PDR). Both reflect the underlying condition of retinal capillary closure, but PDR corresponds to more marked ischaemia, and is characterised by the presence of

NVD or NVE. Advanced ocular ischaemia may also lead to iris neovascularisation.

The prevalence of PDR increases with duration of diabetes. In juvenile onset diabetes, proliferative retinopathy is rare within 10 years of diagnosis, but after 20 years of diabetes it reaches a prevalence of 55%. In maturity onset diabetes PDR is often associated with maculopathy, and may be present at the time the patient is first diagnosed as a diabetic. Again the prevalence of PDR in this group rises with duration to 20% after 20 years in the insulin dependent group. In non-insulin dependent, maturity onset diabetes, PDR is rare. In most instances panretinal laser treatment can prevent the complications of PDR provided that early and sufficient treatment is applied.

NVE nearly always develops from a retinal vein, adjacent to an area of ischaemic retina. Initially the simple vascular channels lie on the surface of the retina but, as they develop and ramify across the retina, they become integrated into the posterior hyaloid face. After a variable period of time the posterior hyaloid may detach. This detachment can be localised to the area of neovascularisation or extend to involve the entire posterior hyaloid. During this process the formerly flat new vessels become elevated, so becoming forward new vessels.

NVD develops in a similar fashion but the stimulus for it to develop requires approximately a quarter of the retina to be ischaemic. Forward new vessels lack the structural support of the adjacent retina and are prone to mechanical disruption. Such forces can produce a cycle of repeated haemorrhage, progressive fibrosis, and contraction. Although some patients present with dense intragel haemorrhages, a less severe bleed may be localised to the retrohyaloid space. In both situations, organisation of the blood can lead to cicatrisation, resulting in tractional retinal detachment. Most diabetic tractional retinal detachments are confined to the posterior pole and have a concave appearance. The exact configuration of the retinal detachment is determined by the resultant vector of anteroposterior and tangential traction, and the extent of the posterior hyaloid detachment.

In diabetic eyes with PDR, the posterior vitreous detachment is limited by the fibrous connections of the posterior hyaloid, the new vessels, and the major retinal vessels. Any forces therefore generated by cicatrisation of the proliferating fibrovascular tissue will be directed to these points of adhesion. If the attachment of the posterior hyaloid is limited, for example, to one small area of retina the tractional retinal detachment will be conical in shape. Conversely, if the posterior hyaloid remains broadly adherent to the retina, any tractional retinal detachment will have a wider base and apex. Some examples of a broadly based tractional detachment are likened to "table top" and "ring" detachments. More complicated configurations of diabetic tractional retinal detachment can occur with persisting retinal ischaemia. For example, if the ischaemia is severe, small atrophic holes may develop in the retina and so convert a tractional detachment into a "combined tractional rhegmatogenous retinal detachment." Introducing a rhegmatogenous element to a pre-existing tractional retinal detachment converts the "tight" concave contour to a more bullous, convex looking detachment It is important to appreciate the differences in contour with "combined retinal detachments" because the atrophic holes are not always obvious. In essence, a "combined tractional rhegmatogenous retinal detachment" is a clear indication for vitrectomy.

In a similar fashion, ongoing retinal ischaemia can induce continuing fibrovascular proliferation. As additional new vessels develop, proliferation occurs along the fibrovascular "scaffold" of the previous generation of new vessels. Complex vector forces can therefore be generated on the pre-existing tractional retinal detachment, if successive generations of fibrovascular tissue contract. Most of the more bizarre tractional retinal detachments are by definition long standing, and have a poor visual prognosis, even with successful vitreoretinal surgery.

Box A   The natural history of progressive retinal ischaemia
Capillary non-perfusion NVE, NVD   Rubeosis iridis Vitreous haemorrhage   Neovascular glaucoma Tractional retinal detachment

Neovascularisation elsewhere

Most NVE develops adjacent to an area of ischaemic retina and arborises across the retina. Although the overall threat to vision is less than for NVD, NVE is also associated with the complications of epiretinal haemorrhage and traction.

The severity of NVE is graded according to the area of neovascularisation, and presence of associated fibrosis, traction, and haemorrhage. Mild NVE is implied when the area of new vessels occupies less than two disc diameters and there are no associated fibrovascular complications. Moderate and severe NVE has correspondingly larger areas of new vessels and increasingly severe associated features.

The presence of retinal ischaemia is a prerequisite for the development of NVE. Conversely, if the ischaemic stimulus is removed or reduced the NVE will involute or show limited growth potential. Spontaneous involution of new vessels is rare, but it is not uncommon to see NVE that remains static over many months or years. Non-progressive NVE is sometimes seen in eyes that have been treated by mild scatter panretinal photocoagulation.

Another type of NVE with limited growth potential is the "raspberry" new vessels (abortive neovascular outgrowths—ANO). These somewhat rare new vessels are associated with a posterior vitreous detachment and tend to remain small and unobtrusive because they are lacking a scaffold. They have a central core of fibrous tissue surrounded by dilated venules which are similar to capillaries and have an appearance like a raspberry. Commonly these "raspberry" new vessels are found in the posterior pole in the area temporal to the fovea inside the arcades, and are closely related to small venules (see figs 3.35–3.37 and 4.14). They project slightly forward from the surface of the retina and may be the cause of small epiretinal haemorrhages. This NVE/ANO is often difficult to treat and may require repeated treatment sessions. It may be a constant cause of subhyaloid or vitreous haemorrhage following an otherwise successful panretinal photocoagulation to NVE or NVD.

The diagnosis of NVE can, on occasion, be difficult, especially when the media are not clear or when the new vessels are small and poorly defined. In most cases the differential diagnosis of NVE can be narrowed down to either intraretinal microvascular anomalies (IRMA) or collaterals. Sometimes the correct diagnosis can be more confidently made by considering the "setting" as well as the clinical features. For example, as collateral vessels develop as a consequence of venous occlusive disease, other features of vein occlusion may be present. Similarly, IRMA develops in response to chronic retinal hypoperfusion and is localised adjacent to ischaemic retinal areas. In some cases where doubt exists, a fluorescein angiogram may be necessary for the correct diagnosis.

Treatment of NVE

Juvenile onset diabetes

The extent of NVE in diabetes can be variable and laser treatment is best titrated according to severity (mild, moderate, or severe). The rare patient with non-insulin dependent, juvenile onset diabetes and mild proliferative disease, such as one or two NVE complexes, can usually be adequately treated without resorting to full scatter panretinal photocoagulation. In most such cases mild NVE can be successfully treated with focal treatment.

Focal laser treatment to NVE

Treatment should be of the area underneath and immediately around the NVE (table 5.1).

Table 5.1 Treatment parameters for treating NVE

Spot size	200–500 µm
Exposure time	0·05–0·2 s
Power	Just to blanch the RPE

Conversely, subjects with insulin dependent juvenile diabetes with moderate or severe NVE formation are best treated with a "modified" or mild scatter panretinal photocoagulation technique. With this treatment option, scatter laser treatment is directed to all areas of capillary non-perfusion in the mid and anterior retina.

Modified panretinal photocoagulation

Treatment should include all areas of capillary non-perfusion (table 5.2).

Table 5.2 Treatment parameters for modified panretinal photocoagulation

Spot size	500 µm
Short exposure time	0·05–0·2 s
Power	Just to blanch the RPE

Adult onset diabetes

NVEs in the adult onset group tend to be less progressive and more responsive to laser treatment than the corresponding lesions in juvenile onset diabetes. If the NVE is limited to a mild or moderate degree, treatment can be limited to the retina immediately around and under the new vessels (focal treatment of NVE) (fig 5.1).

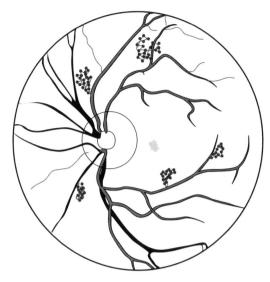

Figure 5.1 Diagrammatic representation of a few small areas of NVE in type II diabetes, where laser treatment can be applied around and under the new vessel complex

Focal and panretinal treatment

In those patients with NVE that is severe, occupying areas of two or three disc diameters, or who have NVE in more than one quadrant, more aggressive laser treatment is required. Most patients with adult onset diabetes and severe peripheral neovascularisation will be successfully controlled with a combination of focal and mild scatter panretinal treatment. This approach combines laser treatment to the area in and around the NVE with additional treatment to the involved quadrant. About 500–800 burns are usually necessary (fig 5.2). This approach also minimises the complication of secondary macular oedema caused by laser induced breakdown of the blood–retina barrier.

Treatment should be by laser directed to the quadrant with the new vessels (table 5.3).

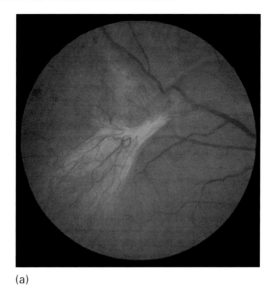

(a)

(b)

Figure 5.2   (a) A neovascular complex in the superotemporal quadrant, with, in addition, some fibrosis following (b) quadrantic scatter photocoagulation and regression of the new vessels

Table 5.3   Treatment parameters for focal and panretinal treatment

Spot size	200–500 μm
Short exposure	0·05–0·2 s
Power	Just to blanch the RPE

Further management of NVE that has already been treated

Both juvenile and late onset diabetic patients need careful follow up after laser treatment. Treated NVE should regress in the first month. If involution does not occur further laser treatment is indicated.

Patients with persistent NVE following focal treatment require further laser treatment under and around the new vessels, with additional panretinal laser applied to the drainage area of the parent vein. This regional approach will be effective in most cases of persistent mild NVE.

Persistent, severe NVE should also be re-treated if satisfactory regression has not occurred within a month.

For patients with juvenile onset diabetes re-treatment involves repeat panretinal photocoagulation. During re-treatment for persistent severe NVE the laser should be aimed at areas between the pre-existing laser burns. This is called a "fill in" approach.

Re-treatment for persistent, severe NVE in type II diabetes is uncommon. If necessary, repeat focal treatment is usually all that is required.

New vessels on the disc

Optic disc neovascularisation in a diabetic subject generally indicates advanced diabetic retinopathy and is an indication for panretinal laser photocoagulation. As with retinal NVE, the stimulus for NVD is retinal ischaemia. It is uncommon to see NVD when the area of retinal capillary non-perfusion is less than a quarter of the total retina.

211

NVD may be derived from the retinal or choroidal circulation, although it is more likely to be from the choroidal circulation if the new vessels originate from the deeper part of the optic cup. It is, however, difficult to be absolutely sure of the exact origin of the new vessels and, for the purposes of management and prognosis, this is immaterial.

In the early stages NVD may be confused with fine, slightly dilated disc capillaries or even small disc collaterals. NVD does not, however, develop in the absence of signs of retinal ischaemia. Alternatively, a fluorescein angiogram may be useful in establishing the diagnosis (see fig 3.38). The subsequent development of new vessels may extend over the surface of the disc and cross the disc margin in one or more quadrants (fig 5.3). There is a propensity for NVD to follow the course of the retinal vessels especially along the temporal arcades. Fibrous tissue accompanies the development of the new vessels and becomes progressively more clinically obvious.

Treatment of NVD

All patients with NVD should be considered for full scatter panretinal photocoagulation. This treatment is a matter of urgency particularly for those with juvenile onset diabetes because NVD not only represents a threat to vision but treatment is more likely to rescue good visual acuity before haemorrhage or fibrosis occurs.

Before treatment the laser operator must familiarise him- or herself with the retinal landmarks, particularly the macular posterior pole features. Many laser operators start treatment in the nasal retina before moving to the temporal quadrants. Others start in the lower half of the retina to finish panretinal treatment in this area before vitreous haemorrhage occurs. A vitreous haemorrhage may be long standing in this region, precluding further photocoagulation.

All four retinal quadrants can be safely treated in the first treatment session. If a 500 μm spot size is used most eyes will require a minimum of 1200 applications for a so called full scatter treatment. Some eyes will only accommodate 1500 burns whereas others will require 3000 burns to cover the retina. The aim of the initial treatment session is to place as many laser applications as possible. It is best to separate each application by the diameter of the spot size used. Care must be taken to avoid the retinal vessels and any area of retinal detachment or fibrosis. Retinal haemorrhages should not be lasered (fig 5.3).

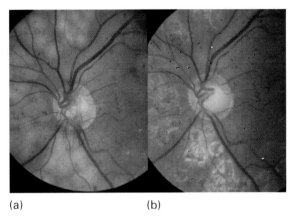

(a)   (b)

Figure 5.3   (a) Retina immediately after laser treatment, showing the gentle laser burns that have been applied for new vessels on the optic disc. (b) Four weeks after treatment there has been complete regression of the neovascular complex

The laser settings are chosen to minimise functional defects. The duration of the burn should be short, between 0·05 and 0·2 s, whereas spot size can vary between 200 and 500 μm, depending on the magnification of the contact lens used. The larger the spot size the fewer the number of burns, although there is less control of burn intensity. The power setting should be continually adjusted to achieve an end point equivalent to a mild blanching of the RPE. Alternatively, the energy density can be modified by defocusing the laser to alter the intensity of the burn. It is important to remember that full thickness retinal burns are not required to achieve involution of new vessels.

Following treatment the patient's central vision is likely to be blurred for up to 10 days. The mechanism of this transient visual disturbance is not clear. Some loss is usually ascribed to a temporary macular oedema and in others is the result of altered accommodation. Permanent changes in colour vision and dark adaptation have been documented following panretinal photocoagulation, although this may remain subclinical.

After treatment the patient should be reassessed 2–4 weeks later. At this time about 50% of patients with NVDs will have undergone complete regression of the neo-vascularisation. NVD that persists after an initial panretinal photocoagulation requires additional treatment directed between the previous laser scars ("fill in") and to the far peripheral retina. A further 1000–1500 burns are easily accommodated. Following this treatment the patient should be reassessed after another 2–4 weeks. Some new vessels can still persist after this treatment and additional "fill in" may be required (fig 5.4). Only a few areas of NVD survive this more extensive treatment regimen. Those eyes may require still more panretinal laser treatment, this time extending treatment to include previously treated areas. Re-treatment is often more painful especially if new burns overlap the existing laser scars. In these patients local anaesthesia may be necessary. On occasion, in highly sensitive people, a retrobulbar anaesthetic may be necessary.

The xenon arc photocoagulator can be used in the management of resistant NVD. As with the laser photocoagulator the xenon arc is tuned to coagulate the retina. A spot size of 4·5° and power setting adjusted to yield a low intensity burn will provide adequate control. Major retinal vessels and areas of detached retina should not be photocoagulated. Secondary macular oedema is more common with the xenon photocoagulator than for the laser but usually resolves within one or two weeks. The oedema is lessened if the number of applications is restricted to 800–1000 burns.

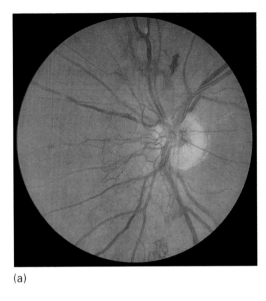

(a)

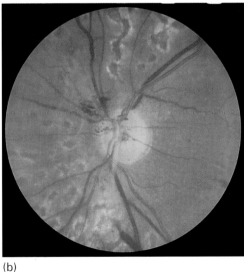

(b)

Figure 5.4 (a–c) Retina showing disc new vessels: the appearance three weeks after treatment with almost complete regression of the new vessels—the treatment was panretinal photocoagulation using 2500+ burns. (d) Three months later, further growth of new vessels had occurred and, in spite of 1500 additional burns, they went on to bleed. (f) Ultimately a further 2000 burns were applied, showing complete regression of the new vessel complex

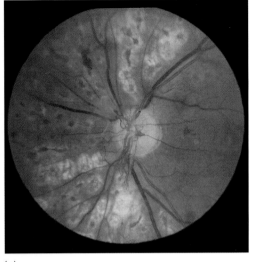

(c)

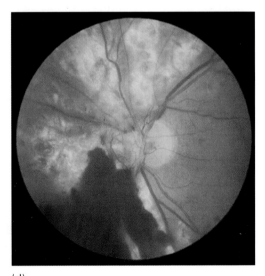

(d)

Figure 5.4 contd

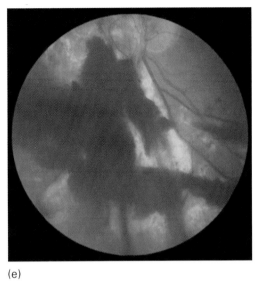

(e)

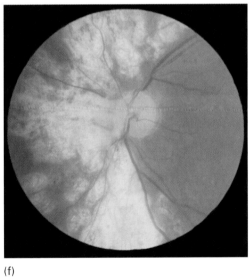

(f)

Figure 5.4   contd

Follow up

Following treatment, new vessels, either NVE or NVD, may persist as thin fine vessels. When seen in the retina they overlie areas of previous photocoagulation. These vessels may be perfused and on fluorescein angiography they may stain or leak minimally. These "ghost vessels" rarely progress and rarely bleed. They may be attached to the posterior vitreous gel or lying "free" in front of the retina or optic disc. On the rare occasions when they do bleed it is usually the result of mechanical forces and the bleeding is minimal. In areas of fibrous tissue new vessels may also persist, and these are usually surrounded by fibrous tissue; on fluorescein angiography they may stain or leak minimally. Once again, they rarely bleed unless exposed to mechanical contraction of the fibrous tissue.

Following satisfactory involution of NVD, appointments should be scheduled in the first year at 4–6 monthly intervals. Subsequent visits can be extended if there is no further evidence of neovascularisation. At each follow up visit the iris, vitreous, and retina should be carefully re-examined. Rubeosis iridis can develop in eyes previously treated with panretinal photocoagulation without recurrent retinal neovascularisation and should be treated before neovascular glaucoma develops. Similarly NVD or NVE can develop in previously treated eyes. In spite of seemingly adequate treatment, some eyes present with recurrent neovascularisation and/or vitreous haemorrhage. If the haemorrhage is small it might be asymptomatic and can be easily overlooked unless the inferior vitreous is surveyed carefully. Blood in the vitreous cavity may be the first evidence of recurrent neovascularisation. Once blood is identified, a careful search of the retina must be undertaken to find the source, and in some patients the new vessels can only be identified by fluorescein angiography.

The visual prognosis for patients following treatment for neovascularisation is good provided that adequate treatment is given before complications develop.

Special management considerations in patients with PDR

1. Persistent new vessels
2. Recurrent new vessels
3. New vessels elsewhere (NVE) and fibrous tissue
4. Vitreous haemorrhage
5. Iris neovascularisation
6. Spontaneous regression
7. New vessels associated with macular oedema
8. Avulsed retinal vessels
9. Choroidal new vessels
10. Pregnancy
11. Cataract

Persistent new vessels

NVE and NVD usually respond well to laser treatment. If involution of the vessels does not occur after full scatter panretinal photocoagulation, a further "fill in" is the first treatment of choice. Closure of NVE by direct treatment is not without risk, and should be limited to the very experienced laser surgeon. This approach should be reserved for persistent new vessels giving rise to recurrent vitreous haemorrhages.

Successful closure of persistent NVE by direct photo-coagulation depends on careful placement of burns along the length of the vessels. The burns are applied from the distal to the proximal end of the new vessel in a contiguous row. The end point is when the laser produces a blanching or darkening of the blood column in the new vessel with interruption of flow. The wavelength of choice for this procedure is dye yellow (577 nm). If the dye laser is not available the blue–green argon laser (488 nm) can be used. The spot size should be sufficient to straddle the new vessel while duration needs to be between 0·2 and 0·5 second. If the desired end point is not reached because of insufficient power, the uptake of the laser energy can be enhanced using a bolus of intravenous fluorescein (0·25–0·5 ml of 20% sodium fluorescein) (figs 5.5 and 5.6). Alternatively, in a two step procedure one can blanch the RPE underneath an NVE and then, using this as a reflective surface, increase the power sufficiently for direct lasering of the new vessel. Not only will some energy be reflected back from the RPE on to the new vessel but the risk of choroidal haemorrhage is greatly reduced.

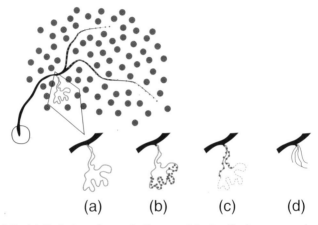

(a)   (b)   (c)   (d)

Figure 5.5 (a) Technique for occluding persistent retinal new vessels that do not overlie a major retinal vein. Previous panretinal photocoagulation or sector coagulation should have been performed, and then the tips of the new vessels are treated (b) and gradually the treatment (c) is extended to the base of the vessel. (d) Once complete occlusion has occurred, then the patient should be re-examined one hour later and re-treated if the vessels reopen. The procedure is repeated until there is permanent closure.

Once the new vessel has been successfully occluded the patient should be re-examined after one hour. In most patients the new vessel will have reopened either in total or in part. In either case re-treatment can be safely performed without further delay to those areas where the vessel is patent. Sometimes following treatment the vessel appears to be more dilated; however, this of course, by having a greater column of blood within the vessel, facilitates additional treatment. During re-treatment the vessel may contract and shorten as

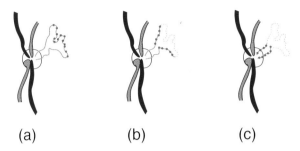

(a)   (b)   (c)

Figure 5.6   Similar technique to that used for disc new vessels is employed for peripheral new vessels

the laser is applied and, on occasion, the whole vascular complex can shrink to the stalk. The closed new vessel should be re-evaluated one hour after any additional re-treatment to ensure that closure is permanent. As a result of the high energies required to close new vessels with direct laser photocoagulation, the presence of pre-existing retinal traction or fibrosis is a contraindication to direct laser treatment. Instead eyes with traction and persistent new vessels should be considered for closed intraocular microsurgery.

Similarly direct treatment to persistent NVEs overlying a retinal vein or the papillomacular bundle should be avoided because of the risk of vitreous haemorrhage.

Recurrent new vessels

All diabetic patients with a history of proliferative retinopathy should be carefully screened for recurrent new vessels. As with primary neovascularisation, recurrent new vessels tend to develop in areas adjacent to sites of non-perfusion. In practice, recurrent NVEs are rarely seen at sites other than the anterior retina or adjacent to pre-existing retinal laser scars.

Recurrent new vessels are usually small and have limited growth potential. Fibrosis and traction are not commonly associated with these new vessels and yet they may be the

221

source of small intermittent vitreous haemorrhages. Control of recurrent NVEs is usually achieved with focal photocoagulation treatment.

NVE and fibrous tissue

If NVE is associated with fibrosis, care should be taken to avoid targeting the laser on the fibrous tissue. At low energy levels, and providing there is no blood or pigment in the fibrous tissue, the light from the laser will not be absorbed. Similarly, low energies should be used when targeting structures adjacent to the fibrous tissue to avoid inducing thermal shrinkage. At high energy levels heat can be conducted to the fibrous tissue and produce a traction retinal detachment. For this reason xenon photocoagulation and retinal cryotherapy are likely to exacerbate fibrous contraction and these treatment modalities should be avoided if possible. Eyes with progressive new vessels within fibrous tissue should be treated with panretinal scatter laser photocoagulation, but if retinal traction approaches the fovea panretinal treatment must be stopped and a vitrectomy should be considered.

In some eyes in spite of full scatter panretinal laser treatment, the new vessels associated with fibrous tissue remain open. The risks of continued proliferation or vitreous haemorrhage in these eyes are, however, significantly less than patent new vessels in untreated eyes. In most cases further "fill in" photocoagulation is not required. If vitreous haemorrhage does occur it is generally limited and reabsorbs within a short period of time.

Vitreous haemorrhage

Vitreous haemorrhage in diabetes indicates the presence of patent new vessels until proved otherwise. Other less common causes of vitreous haemorrhage in the previously treated diabetic eye include recurrent new vessels, avulsed vessels, "raspberry" new vessels, choroidal neovascularisation, contracting fibrous tissue with patent new vessels inside, or associated rhegmatogenous retinal detachment (fig 5.7).

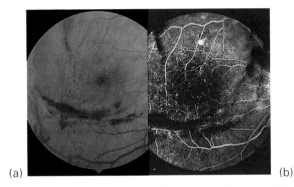

(a)   (b)

Figure 5.7   (a) Preretinal haemorrhage inferiorly placed, although the source of bleeding cannot be identified on clinical examination. (b) Fluorescein angiography, however, reveals a small neovascular complex below the macula, and this clearly is the source of the bleed

In many eyes the source of the vitreous haemorrhage can be determined long before the haemorrhage clears. Even eyes with apparently opaque media can be evaluated with indirect ophthalmoscopy. Bed rest in a head up position will often allow the blood to settle, and help to determine the source of the vitreous haemorrhage. Ultrasonography is useful in those eyes in which retinal detachment may be suspected. If new vessels are suspected but cannot be identified then fluorescein angiography or fluoroscopy may help to find the source of the bleeding.

Iris neovascularisation

Diabetic subjects with extensive retinal capillary non-perfusion can develop iris neovascularisation. Rubeosis iridis typically develops at the pupil margin and extends, sometimes in a skipped pattern, to involve the anterior chamber angle.

Although there are many causes of rubeosis iridis, any diabetic patient presenting with iris neovascularisation should be assumed to have retinal ischaemia until proved otherwise. Full scatter panretinal photocoagulation should be instituted without delay.

Spontaneous regression of new vessels

Spontaneous regression of NVE is uncommon. Some new vessels regress because the ischaemic stimulus has been reduced as a result of retinal atrophy. If regression occurs at a stage before fibrous tissue has become associated with the new vessels, no sequelae of neovascularisation will remain. Conversely, if fibrous tissue develops before the vessels regress a residual grey–white skeletal outline of the vessel will often persist. Ghost vessels are usually only minimally perfused. On fluorescein angiography these vessels do not leak, although the vessel walls may stain. There is no propensity for haemorrhage and no treatment is required.

New vessels associated with macular oedema

The management of patients with both proliferative retinopathy and macular oedema can be difficult because of the cumulative threat to vision. Furthermore, macular oedema may be exacerbated by treating the proliferative retinopathy with panretinal photocoagulation especially in maturity onset diabetes (fig 5.8). Ideally two caveats should govern management:

1 To treat the more immediate threat to vision, commonly the macular oedema
2 If the initial treatment is to the macula, the proliferative retinopathy should be treated in a subsequent treatment session.

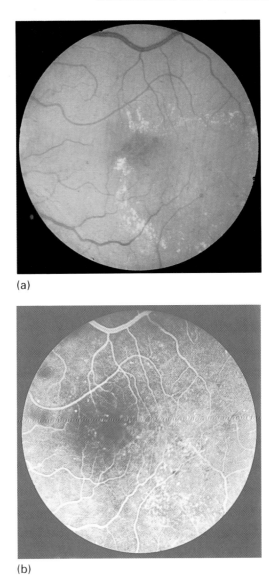

(a)

(b)

Figure 5.8 (a) Large circinate exudate ring; fluorescein angiography in the (b) early and (c) late stages shows considerable leakage from the centre of the circinate ring. (d) NVE some seven years later, (e) the laser scars, and (f) the fluorescein angiogram, showing the recovery in the capillaries and only minimal leakage in the retinal capillaries in the macular area. (g) Appearance some 17 years later, with panretinal photocoagulation and a dry macula; (h) the fluorescein angiogram showing the capillary pattern in the macular area

225

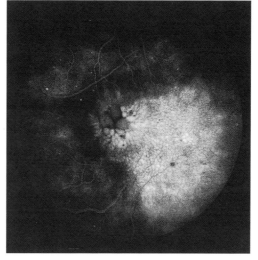

(c)

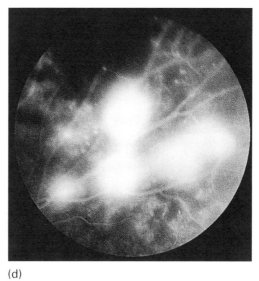

(d)

Figure 5.8   contd

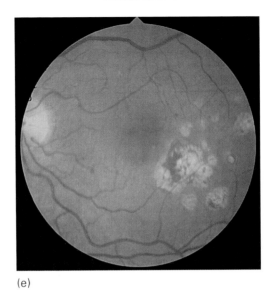

(e)

(f)

Figure 5.8   contd

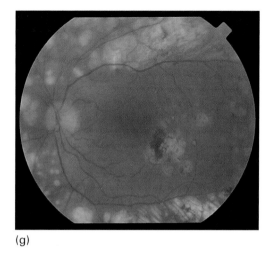

(g)

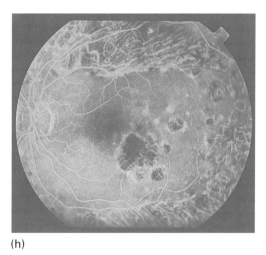

(h)

Figure 5.8   contd

This treatment pattern is a first choice in patients with maturity onset diabetes and macular oedema and new vessels. Most patients can be managed in this way and, unless there is aggressive untreated neovascularisation with vitreous haemorrhage, the macular oedema should be treated first.

An exception to this approach, as has been previously noted, is the young patient with juvenile onset diabetes who has minimal diffuse macular oedema and rapidly accelerating peripheral retinal ischaemia. These patients should be treated initially with panretinal laser treatment. If the macular oedema does not undergo spontaneous resolution, grid treatment can then be applied to the macula.

Avulsed retinal vessels

Detachment of the posterior hyaloid in diabetic patients is sometimes accompanied by avulsion of normal retinal vessels (fig 5.9). In most cases this is asymptomatic, but occasionally avulsion can precipitate a rhegmatogenous retinal detachment or cause recurrent vitreous haemorrhages.

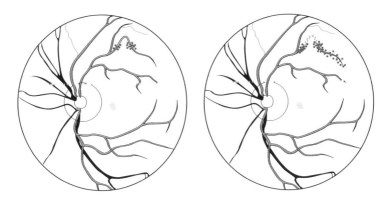

Figure 5.9 Diagrammatic representation of the management of recurrently bleeding avulsed vessels. Initially laser treatment should be applied at the base of the vessel, and then subsequently along the vessel itself; if this fails to stop the recurrent bleeding, then the vessel can be closed off

The development of a retinal hole in an area of traction retinal detachment has sinister implications and may lead to a total retinal detachment. Most cases require treatment with closed intraocular microsurgery.

Recurrent vitreous haemorrhages from avulsed retinal vessels are usually small and do not require treatment unless they become frequent or disabling. In most instances permanent closure of the avulsed portion is required to prevent ongoing haemorrhages. If the media are clear, direct laser photocoagulation to the offending vessel is the treatment of choice. To facilitate closure it is best to pre-treat the distal attached portion of the vessel with laser photocoagulation. Vasospasm in this segment will reduce overall blood flow and enhance uptake in the avulsed portion.

Choroidal new vessels

Choroidal new vessels are an uncommon complication of laser treatment. Typically they develop in heavily or re-treated areas of retina. Initially the choroidal new vessels are small and usually confined to the base of the treatment scar. Some extend with time but their growth potential is limited and it is rare to find choroidal new vessels emerging beyond the treated area.

Treatment to choroidal new vessels is not required unless central vision is threatened or the vessels become a source of recurrent vitreous haemorrhages. Successful closure of these vessels by laser photocoagulation is difficult because of the limited uptake resulting from the lack of adjacent pigment. Direct closure of the vessels can be attempted although a combination of this approach and additional laser burns around the photocoagulation scar may be necessary.

Pregnancy

In pregnancy, patients with moderate or severe NPDR may progress rapidly to PDR. The cause for this progression is uncertain and this does not occur in all pregnant women. Women most vulnerable include primigravidas, and those with renal impairment and/or arterial hypertension.

It is unusual to see progression of retinopathy before week 16 of pregnancy but all pregnant diabetic women should be reviewed early in the first trimester. If diabetic retinopathy is present, repeat examinations should be conducted at one month intervals until delivery. Conversely those women without retinopathy need only be reviewed on a two monthly basis. During the second trimester capillary closure can be rapid. In most cases the clinical signs of a proliferative retinopathy are obvious and early panretinal treatment is indicated. It is important to ensure that the treatment is adequate and most will require full scatter panretinal laser treatment and additional "fill in" sessions.

The presence of progressive new vessels does not preclude vaginal delivery but delivery by this route may be safer with an assisted delivery. Close liaison with the woman's obstetrician is essential in the later stages of gestation especially if induction is planned before term.

It is uncommon to see progressive retinopathy in multigravid women but continued ophthalmic observation is suggested for all pregnant diabetic women. If successful panretinal photocoagulation has already been carried out, there is a minimal risk of recurrence of the proliferative process with pregnancy.

In some pregnant diabetic women diffuse macular oedema occurs with variable but possibly profound visual loss. The oedema often resolves spontaneously after delivery and only persists in a minority. Focal laser treatment should, however, be performed when macular oedema is "clinically significant."

Cataract

Cataracts are a major cause of visual morbidity in the diabetic population. Furthermore, they can preclude an adequate examination of the retina and make photocoagulation of diabetic retinopathy difficult. Conversely, not all cataracts need extraction and, providing that the visual

231

requirements are met and the retina can be surveyed, intervention can be delayed.

The incorporation of a laser with an indirect ophthalmoscope has simplified treatment of some diabetic patients with media opacities. The lens opacities not only degrade the view of the fundus, but scatter and absorb energy during photocoagulation. Absorption is worst with those eyes that have yellowing of the crystalline lens whereas light scatter is worse with a blue–green laser. Longer wavelength lasers are affected less by media opacities.

The preferred method of cataract extraction in a diabetic eye is by the extracapsular or phacoemulsification technique including small incisions. An intraocular lens is not contraindicated and indeed provides the best method of providing visual rehabilitation. We prefer a lens implant with a large diameter of 6·5 mm which facilitates subsequent panretinal photocoagulation or vitrectomy. Cataract extraction in itself may cause deterioration of untreated macular oedema, PDR, and iris neovascularisation. Therefore, as long as the cataract is not too dense, photocoagulation of the retina should be carried out first, and the cataract extraction should be delayed until retinopathy is stabilised and rubeosis iridis has regressed. If a dense cataract precludes photocoagulation, laser therapy should be performed during or immediately following cataract surgery. Small tunnel incisions are very stable and allow the application of a contact lens within a few days (figs 5.10–5.14).

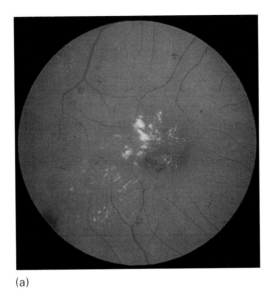

(a)

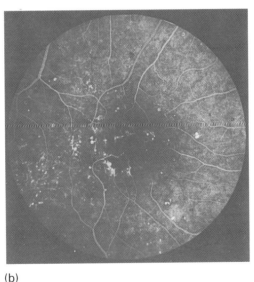

(b)

Figure 5.10   This case illustrates many of the long term problems associated with diabetic retinopathy and is shown in figs 5.10–5.14. (a–d) Initially this patient was seen in 1977 when she first presented. The patient was an insulin dependent diabetic woman, who after 15 years of diabetes presented with rubeotic glaucoma in her left eye and diabetic CSMO associated with moderate proliferative retinopathy. Fluorescein angiography confirmed the leakage in the posterior pole, associated with dilatation of the retinal capillaries.

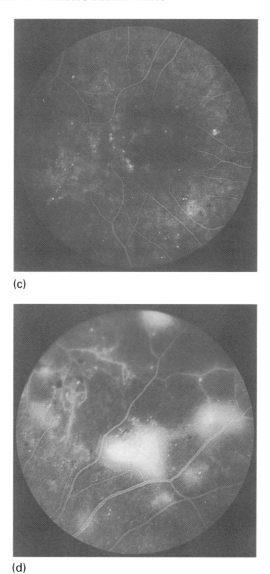

(c)

(d)

Figure 5.10 contd—(d) The peripheral fluorescein angiogram shows capillary closure with neovascularisation. She was considered a high risk patient, had a small amount of laser applied to the macula, and panretinal photocoagulation applied to the peripheral retina

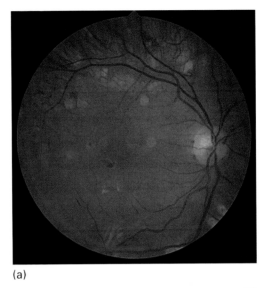

(a)

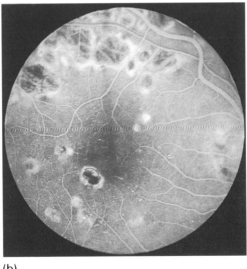

(b)

Figure 5.11   The same patient in 1986, showing regression of the retinal new vessels and improvement in the appearance of the macula with absorption of the exudates and return of the retinal macular capillaries to a more normal appearance. At this visit the patient had a small vitreous haemorrhage and it was possible, on clinical examination, to find the source of this haemorrhage; the fluorescein angiogram (c), however, shows a small new vessel temporal to the macula. This was successfully lasered and there was resolution of the haemorrhage

235

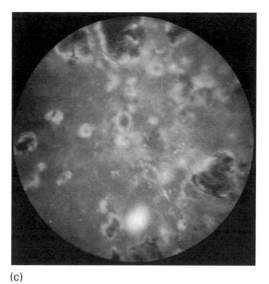

(c)

Figure 5.11 contd

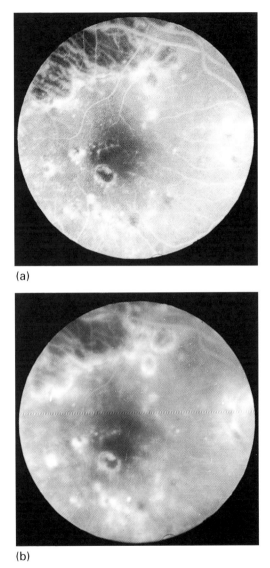

(a)

(b)

Figure 5.12 (a–c) In 1994, the same patient had slow progressive loss of vision as a result of development of a cataract, and cataract extraction was carried out in March 1994, with intraoperative fluorescein angiography. This showed at the time of surgery that there was dilatation and leakage from the paramacular capillaries and the posterior pole. (d–g) The patient was then seen again four days after the cataract operation and fluorescein angiography was again carried out, showing persistence of the dilatation and some leakage in the posterior pole

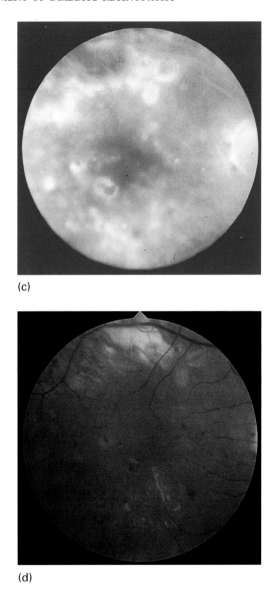

(c)

(d)

Figure 5.12   contd

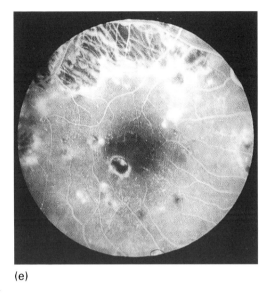

(e)

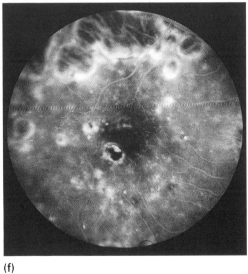

(f)

Figure 5.12   contd

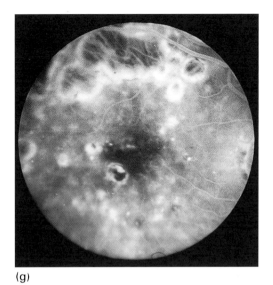

(g)

Figure 5.12 contd

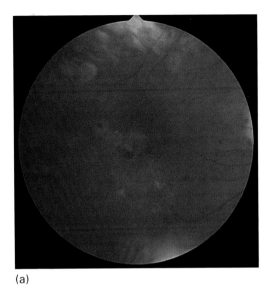

(a)

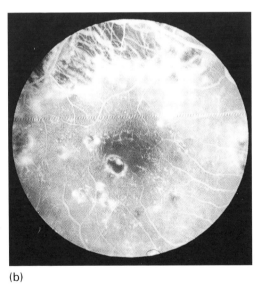

(b)

Figure 5.13 (a–d) Two months after cataract extraction, a similar appearance was obtained and (e–h) some four months after cataract extraction there was still some slight dilatation, although the capillaries were beginning to recover

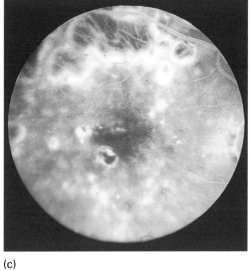

(c)

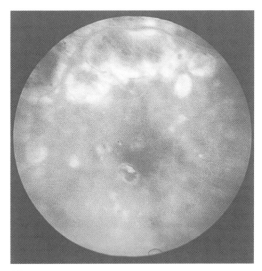

(d)

Figure 5.13   contd

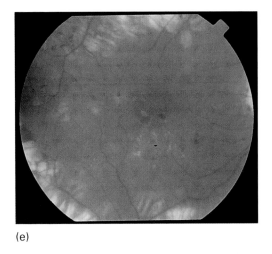

(e)

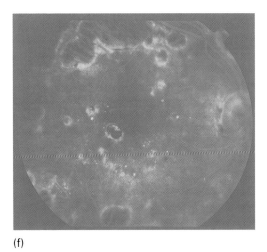

(f)

Figure 5.13 contd

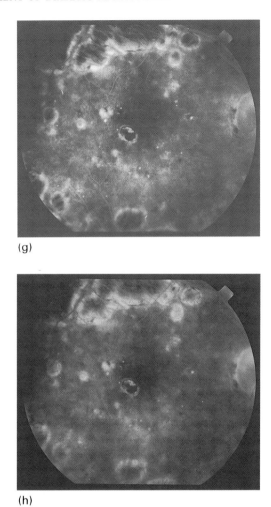

(g)

(h)

Figure 5.13 contd

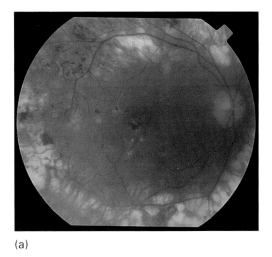

(a)

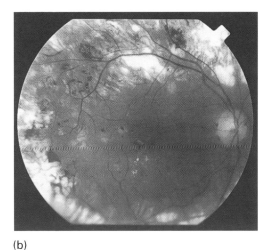

(b)

Figure 5.14 (a–e) Six months after surgery, there was a return of the capillaries in the posterior pole, to their precataract appearance, and at this time the visual acuity had stabilised. This case therefore illustrates the effect of peripheral treatment on macular capillaries, the possible need for fluorescein angiography to identify bleeding new vessels, the effect of cataract extraction on macular capillaries, and the effect that occurs at the time of surgery. It also shows the long drawn out period for recovery of the macular capillaries

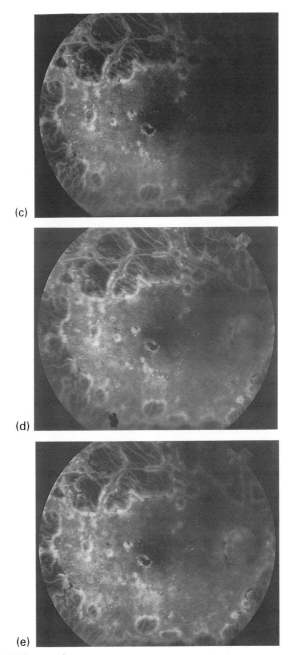

(c)

(d)

(e)

Figure 5.14   contd

444

Management of advanced PDR

Vitrectomy

There are patients with PDR in whom full scatter panretinal photocoagulation is carried out too late or is not sufficient to prevent ongoing proliferation and formation of non-clearing vitreous haemorrhage. If a vitreous haemorrhage does not clear spontaneously within 2–3 months allowing further photocoagulation, vitrectomy should not be delayed and immediate panretinal endophotocoagulation is needed. Early vitrectomy has proved to be a useful technique to prevent blindness in these eyes. It is mandatory in these cases not to delay panretinal laser treatment further. With improved modern vitrectomy techniques, such as *en bloc* delamination of epiretinal membranes, it is possible to improve vision in 70% of eyes. The updated indications for vitrectomy in diabetic retinopathy are given in box B. With improvement

---

Box B Indications for vitrectomy in diabetic retinopathy

- Non-clearing vitreous haemorrhage
- Severe proliferative retinopathy not responding to adequate laser treatment
- Macular detachment
- Tractional detachment threatening the macula
- Combined tractional and rhegmatogenous detachment
- Dense premacular haemorrhage not resolving in spite of YAG laser treatment of the inner limiting membrane
- Recurrent "deposits" behind intraocular lens
- Cataract preventing photocoagulation
- Iris neovascularisation and vitreous haemorrhage
- Anterior hyaloidal fibrovascular proliferation
- Macular oedema with vitreous traction
- Ghost cell glaucoma not controlled with medical treatment
- Fibrinous reaction with retinal detachment

in surgical technique and the introduction of intraocular tamponading agents such as heavy liquid, gas, and silicone oil, there has been a change in the indications for vitrectomy. Twenty years ago most vitrectomies were performed for non-clearing vitreous haemorrhage; today the most common reason for surgical interference is tractional retinal detachment involving the fovea. This may well reflect the improved results of advanced laser management of diabetic retinopathy with time.

If a full scatter panretinal photocoagulation with a minimum 1200 exposures has been performed before vitreous haemorrhage occurred, it is possible to wait for three months for clearing of the vitreous gel. By contrast, if B scan ultrasonography reveals tractional retinal detachment or progressive neovascularisation emerging from the optic disc (NVD), early vitrectomy must be considered. If the macula is involved in tractional retinal detachment, vitrectomy must be performed immediately or the prognosis for final visual outcome fades. If traction to the fovea is long standing, cystoid macular oedema may evolve which is often irreversible and does not respond to focal or grid photocoagulation. Also patients with insulin dependent type I diabetes should undergo vitrectomy earlier than those with type II as a result of the more aggressive progression of proliferative activity in these young patients.

If vitrectomy is performed, it is mandatory to remove the vitreous gel completely. The vitreous base must be removed in particular with great care, using an indentation technique to prevent anterior hyaloid fibrovascular proliferation. If cataract and vitreous haemorrhage are present at the same time, a combined procedure, including tunnel incision, phacoemulsification, vitrectomy, and endolaser photocoagulation, is most effective. The most complicated situation is combined tractional and rhegmatogenous retinal detachment. Commonly small retinal breaks exist alongside epiretinal proliferation. These breaks are often difficult to detect and may only become obvious during vitrectomy. Epiretinal membranes must be removed completely and coagulation of new vessel stalks is essential. On occasion, retinal traction can only be released by retinotomy, and then an intraocular tamponade such as gas or silicone oil is needed. As a rule silicone oil should never be applied to fibrous tissue and remaining epiretinal membranes.

Another common risk factor for deterioration is with young diabetic patients who have large premacular or recurrent subhyaloidal haemorrhages which take a long time to reabsorb and may preclude further panretinal photo-coagulation. In these eyes the preretinal haemorrhage may act as a scaffold for underlying new vessels. To wait for spon-taneous clearing of premacular subhyaloid haemorrhage means taking a high risk of fibrous scar formation and permanent visual loss (see fig 3.9). Opening of the inner limiting membrane with the Nd:YAG laser and allowing the entrapped blood to drain into the vitreous gel is successful in most cases, but may not work if the haemorrhage is long standing and already organised. In these cases only vitrectomy can restore vision.

Iris neovascularisation in the presence of vitreous haemorrhage is also a reason for immediate surgical interference. Whereas in the early days of vitrectomy, rubeosis iridis was considered a contraindication for vitrectomy, it is well recognised now that early removal of the vitreous haemorrhage and panretinal endophotocoagulation both offer the best chances in such eyes. Surgical removal of posterior synechiae and membranes may also help to control intraocular pressure. If an additional cataract is present it should be removed during the same procedure, because the high risk of cataract surgery in the presence of untreated PDR, including iris neovascularisation and poor visual outcome, is now well recognised.

The diagnosis of so called "ghost cell glaucoma" in the presence of vitreous haemorrhage should only be established if no other underlying reason for the elevated intraocular pressure can be diagnosed. In ghost cell glaucoma red blood cells are washed forward into the anterior chamber and there they block the outflow in the trabecular meshwork.

Performing standard three port vitrectomy and rinsing the vitreous cavity can improve the situation. In essence, the prognosis following vitreoretinal surgery in diabetes depends on the grade of previous retinal and optic nerve damage, and the quality and quantity of preoperative laser treatment (box C).

Box C   Predisposing factors for poor visual outcome after vitrectomy in PDR

- Previously no or inadequate photocoagulation
- Optic nerve atrophy
- Either ischaemic or extensive exudative maculopathy
- Delayed vitrectomy

Iris neovascularisation and secondary glaucoma

If PDR is not adequately treated with panretinal photocoagulation, iris neovascularisation may evolve. Iris neovascularisation usually starts at the pupil margins as fine curly rubeosis iridis. In advanced stages there is membrane formation which may reach into the anterior chamber angle and block the trabecular meshwork. As a result intraocular pressure rises and finally secondary glaucoma may lead to optic atrophy and a painful eye. Untreated this neovascular glaucoma leads to blindness and finally phthisis bulbi.

Pharmacological treatment

- β Blockers
- Adrenergic drugs
- Steroids
- Carbonic anhydrase inhibitors

The most important measure to treat developing rubeosis iridis is to perform full scatter panretinal photocoagulation which may lead to fibrosis and regression of iris neo-vascularisation. This can be difficult to perform as a result of corneal oedema and anterior fibrinous uveitis. Therefore, initially the elevated intraocular pressure and the associated anterior segment inflammation have to be treated. Topical steroids, β-adrenergic blockers, and adrenergic eye drops are helpful in controlling this situation. Carbonic anhydrase inhibitors are also indicated if the intraocular pressure is not controlled by topical treatment. Adrenergic eye drops also cause constriction of the new vessels in the anterior chamber angle and are helpful in dilating the pupil for laser treatment.

Cyclodestructive procedures

- Cyclocryocoagulation
- Nd:YAG: contact/non-contact cyclophotocoagulation
- Diode laser: contact/non-contact cyclophoto-coagulation (CPC)

If pharmacological treatment does not succeed in controlling intraocular pressure, cyclodestructive procedures are the method of choice. Cyclocryotherapy is still used in most centres and causes a sufficient hypotensive effect, although it is associated with a relatively high risk of phthisis bulbi. Recently Nd:YAG cyclophotocoagulation, in either contact or non-contact mode, has become the method of choice by a number of ophthalmologists because of better titration of dosage and reduced risk of phthisis bulbi. There are two treatment patterns:

1 Application of 20 exposures over 180°
2 Application of 40 exposures over 360°.

The usual energy applied varies from 3·5 up to 7 joules in the free running mode with a short exposure time of 20 ms, and the burns are placed 1·5 mm behind the limbus on the scleral side. Some laser operators prefer to use a Shield's cyclophotocoagulation contact lens; others apply these exposures without a contact lens. The major advantage of the contact lens is to compress the conjunctival blood vessels. The advantage of the 180° treatment pattern is a relatively mild inflammatory response and a rather low incidence of early postoperative rise in intraocular pressure. The 360° pattern technique has a more marked hypotensive effect, but also more pronounced non-therapeutic side effects such as hypopyon, hyphaema, and anterior fibrinous uveitis. All these complications can be controlled easily by topical steroids. All these cyclodestructive treatments need to be carried out under retrobulbar anaesthesia.

The continuous wave diode laser emitting in the near infrared at 810 nm also has properties of good transmission through the sclera. There are, as with the Nd:YAG laser, non-contact as well as contact delivery systems using a special fibreoptic probe (IRIS Medical, G-Probe). With the non-contact delivery system via a slitlamp microscope, targeting at 1·5 mm behind the limbus means very precise location of burns. Up to 100 exposures with 1·5 W and 1·5 s duration can be applied to the ciliary body. There is significant lowering of intraocular pressure, and there are no conjunctival burns except in black patients with a highly pigmented conjunctiva. These rather low powered effects cause very little inflammatory response of the eye.

Using high power diode lasers with a maximum output of 2 W and a special fibreoptic probe for delivery in the contact mode improves trans-scleral transmission considerably. Clinical studies have shown instant and effective lowering of intraocular pressure. The final rate of phthisis bulbi with this method is below that of cyclocryotherapy.

Filtering and drainage surgery

- Trabeculectomy followed by a cyclodestructive procedure
- Trabeculectomy including antimetabolite drugs
- Molteno Seton implant

In many cases of diabetic neovascular glaucoma a reduction of intraocular pressure is required instantly, and there may be no time to await the intraocular pressure lowering effects of a cyclodestructive procedure. Formerly, neovascularisation in the anterior chamber angle and trabecular meshwork was regarded as a contraindication for trabeculectomy in such eyes. Therefore trabeculectomy was only performed in situations where immediate reduction of intraocular pressure was essential; consecutive scarring of the filtering bleb was counteracted by a subsequent cyclodestructive procedure. The cyclodestructive procedure then provided a hypotensive effect when the filtering channel was obliterated. With this treatment regimen it is often possible to overcome situations with instant severe elevation of intraocular pressure. Subsequent regression of corneal oedema allows access to further panretinal treatment which is facilitated using the laser indirect ophthalmoscope.

Intraoperative application of antimetabolite drugs such as mitomycin C is possibly replacing Molteno Seton implants. Pilot studies have shown positive results and there now may be a new perspective for filtering surgery in the treatment of neovascular glaucoma.

Diabetic cataract

Cataracts are a well recognised complication of diabetes mellitus. It has been shown that about 20% of all cataract extractions carried out in the United Kingdom are performed on diabetic patients, whereas only 3% of the British population are diabetic. Accelerated formation of diabetic cataracts results from the accumulation of glycosylation products in the lens at an earlier age than in non-diabetic subjects. These cataracts are similar to the age related cataracts but occur at a much younger age. The types of cataracts occurring in most diabetic patients are cortical cataracts and, in a minority, posterior subcapsular cataracts. In uncontrolled ketotic diabetic patients, an unusually rapid cataract may develop within a period of a few hours which results in the snow flake cataract. This rare type of cataract may occur as a result of a sudden increase in fluid caused by the hyperosmolarity of the lens.

Cataract extraction

The procedure of choice for cataract extraction in diabetic individuals is by the extracapsular route or phacoemulsification technique. Although previously controversial, there is now no contraindication to the use of a posterior chamber lens implant. A large optic PMMA lens of 6·5 mm diameter facilitates visualisation of the retina, so future panretinal laser treatment and vitrectomy should become necessary. The use of the self sealing tunnel incision is particularly useful if combined cataract extraction and vitrectomy is needed. In those eyes in which there is no view of the retina as the result of a dense cataract, ultrasonography is indicated before cataract extraction, and assessment of the pupillary reaction for an afferent defect is essential. If retinopathy is suspected, early visualisation with possible laser treatment is required and early assessment within a day or so of cataract surgery should be carried out. It is also possible to perform indirect ophthalmoscopy at the time of surgery before the insertion of the intraocular lens implant to assess the presence of retinopathy so as to plan future therapy. In cases with high risk proliferative retinopathy or marked rubeosis iridis, it is possible to carry out panretinal photocoagulation during cataract surgery using the laser indirect ophthalmoscope before insertion of the intraocular lens implant. This may result in a more stable postoperative retinal situation, avoiding possible rapid progression of PDR. In diabetic subjects the postoperative course can be fairly stormy with a proportion of cases developing fibrinous anterior uveitis. The pre-operative and postoperative use of steroids in diabetic patients may modify this complication.

Cataract extraction has been shown to cause progression of macular oedema, proliferative retinopathy, and even the precipitation of a vitreous haemorrhage. Early recognition and treatment may modify the course. The rate of posterior capsule opacification is as common in the eyes of diabetic individuals as it is in the non-diabetic eye; if Nd:YAG laser capsulotomy is required, this should be made as large as possible to aid visualisation and panretinal treatment of the retina.

Cataract extraction may cause aggravation of existing rubeosis iridis, particularly if the posterior capsule is ruptured at the time of surgery. It is unusual to see advancement of rubeosis iridis secondary to a Nd:YAG laser capsulotomy. In cases of iris capture the rubeosis may spread from the pupil margin on to the posterior capsule and extend across the anterior surface of the posterior capsule. This is called rubeosis capsulare. Iris neovascularisation may also extend through dialling holes of the intraocular lens implant on to the anterior surface of the posterior capsule. Thus intraocular implants with dialling holes should be avoided. New vessels may also extend across the posterior surface of the capsule emerging from the peripheral ischaemic retina, growing along the anterior hyaloidal face, avoiding the ciliary processes but finally reaching the centre of the posterior capsule. This has been described as anterior hyaloidal fibrovascular proliferation.

It is essential in diabetic patients with retinopathy in which there is visualisation of the retina to carry out adequate laser treatment for either macular oedema or proliferative retinopathy before performing cataract extraction. If we define a visual acuity of 6/12 or better as a successful outcome in patients after cataract extraction, then in non-diabetic patients the target of 6/12 or better is achieved in about 95%

of patients. In diabetic patients without retinopathy that same target figure can be achieved. Once retinopathy has developed, and with increasing severity of retinopathy, the visual success rate drops considerably. The worst results are in those with active proliferative disease.

The best results are obtained in those who have no retinopathy, NPDR, no clinically significant macular oedema, or quiescent proliferative retinopathy. Those with macular oedema and active PDR have the worst visual outcome. Clearly photocoagulation treatment at an early opportunity before cataract extraction should be performed, although once the adequate view of the retina is lost, cataract extraction is essential.

Appendix I

Screening for diabetic retinopathy

Diabetic retinopathy is the only blinding ocular disease in which severe visual loss really can be avoided by retinal photocoagulation, provided that the screening, the indications, and the treatment patterns are well done. This is in contrast to other blinding ocular disease such as age related macular degeneration or glaucoma, in which laser treatment plays a less beneficial role.

Potentially blinding lesions of diabetic retinopathy, such as proliferative NVD/NVE or clinically significant macular oedema (CSMO), may develop a long time before the patient realises any visual deterioration. By contrast, when the patient realises visual deterioration the fundus lesion may be well advanced and laser treatment may come too late. To avoid such delay and unnecessary severe visual loss, screening for diabetic retinopathy is required on a regular basis. The screening intervals depend on the duration of diabetes, the age of the patient, the type of diabetes (juvenile onset, maturity onset), and the grade of diabetic retinopathy at the last visit. In addition, there are special situations such as pregnancy.

Screening for diabetic retinopathy requires an assessment of the best corrected visual acuity, a slitlamp examination, and stereoscopic biomicroscopy of the fundus in mydriasis to detect retinal thickening and proliferation.

Children

In diabetic children, diabetic retinopathy is rare before puberty and lesions that require laser treatment never develop before that time. Therefore diabetic children should be screened for retinopathy from puberty onwards once a year until mild non-proliferative diabetic retinopathy (NPDR) develops. Then they should be looked at every six months because, even in eyes with mild NPDR, a CSMO may develop. Once severe NPDR has developed the follow up examination should be performed every three months because now neovascularisation may develop and mild scatter panretinal treatment may become necessary.

Juvenile onset diabetes

Patients with juvenile onset diabetes should be screened once a year starting with year 8 after the diagnosis of an insulin dependent diabetes mellitus has been made. Once mild NPDR has developed, continue as described for diabetic children. The special considerations for pregnant women are given elsewhere in this book.

Maturity onset diabetes

The problem with this group of diabetic patients is that you never know when these patients became diabetic. Therefore you have to screen the fundus immediately after the diagnosis was made. If no retinopathy is present, an examination once a year is sufficient. Once mild NPDR has developed, the eyes should be examined twice a year with special emphasis on diabetic macular oedema. If more severe retinopathy develops, this regimen should be tightened to a quarterly basis.

The St Vincent Declaration*

Representatives of Government Health Departments and patients' organisations from all European countries met with diabetes experts under the aegis of the Regional Offices of the World Health Organization and the International Diabetes Federation in St Vincent, Italy on October 10–12 1989. The following recommendations were agreed upon and it was urged that they should be presented in all countries throughout Europe for implementation.

General goals for people—children and adults—with diabetes

- Sustained improvement in health experience and a life approaching normal expectations in quality and quantity.
- Prevention and cure of diabetes and of its complications by intensifying research effort.

Five year targets

- Elaborate, initiate, and evaluate comprehensive programmes for detection and control of diabetes and of its complications with self care and community support as major components.
- Raise awareness in the population and among health care professionals of the present opportunities and the future needs for prevention of the complications of diabetes and of diabetes itself.
- Organise training and teaching in diabetes management and care for people of all ages with diabetes, for their families, friends, and working associates, and for the health care team.

* Source: Diabetes mellitus in Europe: A problem at all ages in all countries. A model for prevention and self care. St Vincent (Italy), 10–12 October 1989. A meeting organised by WHO and IDF in Europe. (Diabetes Care and Research in Europe. The St Vincent Declaration. *Diabetic Medicine* 1990;7:360.)

- Ensure that care for children with diabetes is provided by individuals and teams specialised in the management of both diabetes and children, and that families with a diabetic child get the necessary social, economic, and emotional support.
- Reinforce existing centres of excellence in diabetes care, education, and research. Create new centres where the need and potential exist.
- Promote independence, equity, and self sufficiency for all people with diabetes—children, adolescents, those in the working years of life, and elderly people.
- Remove hindrances to the fullest possible integration of the diabetic citizen into society.
- Implement effective measures for the prevention of costly complications by: reducing new blindness caused by diabetes by one third or more; reducing numbers of people entering end stage diabetic renal failure by at least one third; reducing by one half the rate of limb amputations for diabetic gangrene; cutting morbidity and mortality from coronary heart disease in the diabetic patient by vigorous programmes of risk factor education; and achieving pregnancy outcome in the diabetic woman that approximates that of the non-diabetic woman.
- Establish monitoring and control systems using state of the art information technology for quality assurance of diabetes health care provision, and for laboratory and technical procedures in diabetes diagnosis, treatment, and self management.
- Promote European and international collaboration in programmes of diabetes research and development through national, regional, and WHO agencies, and in active partnership with diabetes patients' organisations.
- Take urgent action in the spirit of the WHO programme "Health for All," to establish joint machinery between WHO and IDF, European Region, to initiate, accelerate, and facilitate the implementation of these recommendations.

A protocol for screening for diabetic retinopathy in Europe*

Protocol for screening for diabetic eye complications

- Identification and collection of clinical data
- Onset of visual symptoms
- History of glaucoma
- Measurement of visual acuity unaided and, if necessary, with spectacles and/or pinhole
- Pupil dilatation with 2·5–10% phenylephrine and/or 1% tropicamide and/or 1% cyclopentolate eye drops
- Lens examination for cataract with +10 lens in ophthalmoscopy or red reflex photography
- Fundus examination.

Method for fundus examination

Two readily available techniques can be used for retinal examination: ophthalmoscopy and fundus photography.

What is being looked for?

Sight threatening retinopathy, requiring immediate referral

Proliferative
New vessels on the optic disc or elsewhere in the retina
Preretinal haemorrhage
Fibrous tissue

Advanced diabetic eye disease
Vitreous haemorrhage
Fibrous tissue
Recent retinal detachment
Rubeosis iridis

* Source: Retinopathy Working Party. *Diabetic Medicine* 1991;**8**:262–7.

Lesions to be referred for assessment as soon as possible by an ophthalmologist

---

Pre-proliferative retinopathy
 Venous irregularities (beading, reduplication, loops)
 Multiple haemorrhages
 Multiple cotton wool spots
 Intraretinal microvascular abnormalities (IRMA)

Non-proliferative retinopathy with macular involvement
 Reduced visual acuity not corrected by pinhole
  (suggestive of macular oedema)
 Haemorrhages and/or hard exudates within one disc
  diameter of the macula, with or without visual
  loss

Non-proliferative retinopathy without macular involvement
 Large circinate or plaque exudates within the major
  temporal vascular arcades

Any other reasonable findings that the observer
cannot interpret with reasonable certainty

The following lesions can be followed up in the screening clinic 6–12 months later:

Non-proliferative retinopathy
 Cotton wool spots in small numbers not associated
  with pre-proliferative lesions
 Occasional haemorrhages and/or microaneurysms
  ("red dots and blots") and hard exudates not
  within one disc diameter of the macular area
 Drusen may sometimes be confused with hard
  exudates; if not associated with other signs of age
  related macular degeneration, they are not
  considered important

Who should screen?

- Ideally ophthalmologists
- Train more specialists in diagnosis of diabetic retinopathy
- Doctor in charge of diabetic patient should be responsible for organisation of screening when not feasible for ophthalmologist to screen
- Health care providers trained for screening with the proviso that their ability is evaluated first
- If medical photographers carry out retinal photography, then experienced readers should evaluate the pictures.

When to screen?

- At onset of puberty
- After puberty, eyes should be examined at diagnosis, at least two yearly thereafter, and at least annually if retinopathy appears

Data collected

Outcome of previous screening session (treatment YES/NO)
Visual acuity
No retinopathy
Non-proliferative retinopathy not requiring referral
Non-proliferative retinopathy requiring referral
Macular involvement
Pre-proliferative retinopathy
Proliferative retinopathy
Photocoagulated proliferative retinopathy
Advanced diabetic disease
Legal blindness
Other eye disease (specify)

- More frequent examinations are necessary if there is any intercurrent illness or renal impairment
- Before conception (if possible), at confirmation of pregnancy, and every three months, or more frequently if necessary
- Defaulters should be examined immediately.

A leaflet has been prepared for distribution to patients and also diabetic retinopathy screening cards are available.

Appendix II

Flow charts of classification and management of diabetic retinopathy

Classification of diabetic retinopathy

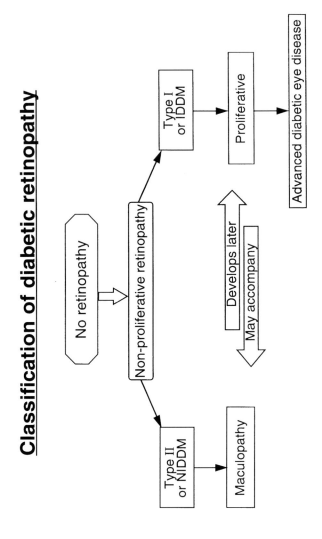

Management of non-proliferative retinopathy

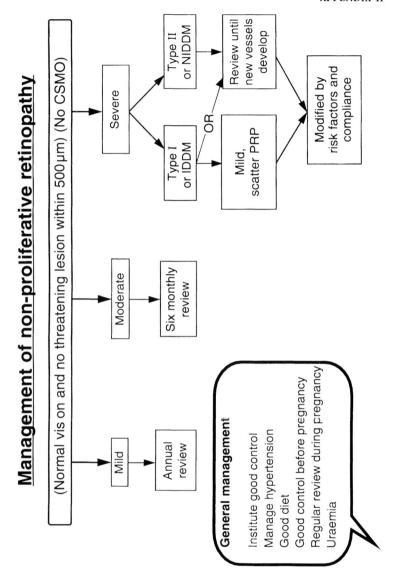

(Normal vis on and no threatening lesion within 500 μm) (No CSMO)

Mild → Annual review

Moderate → Six monthly review

Severe → Type I or IDDM / Type II or NIDDM

Type II or NIDDM → Review until new vessels develop

Type I or IDDM → Mild, scatter PRP OR Review until new vessels develop

→ Modified by risk factors and compliance

General management

Institute good control
Manage hypertension
Good diet
Good control before pregnancy
Regular review during pregnancy
Uraemia

Classification of maculopathy

Management of maculopathy

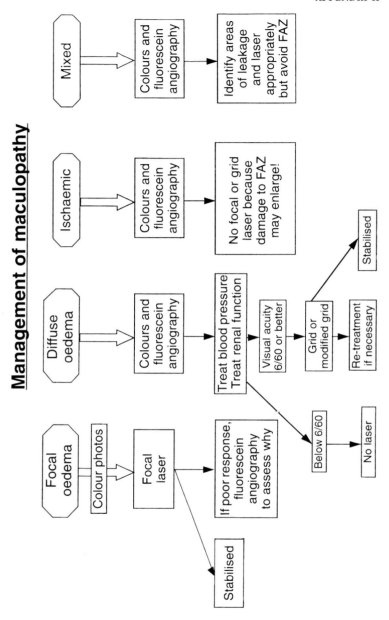

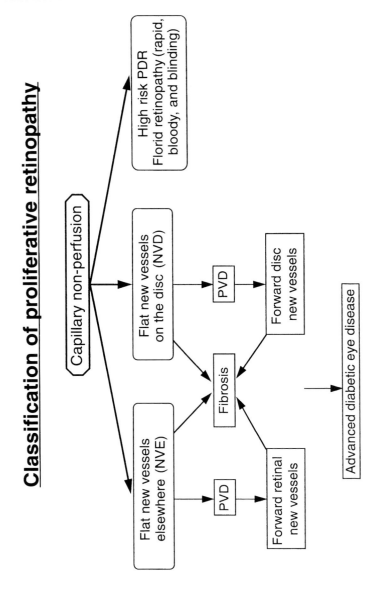

Classification of proliferative retinopathy

Management of proliferative retinopathy

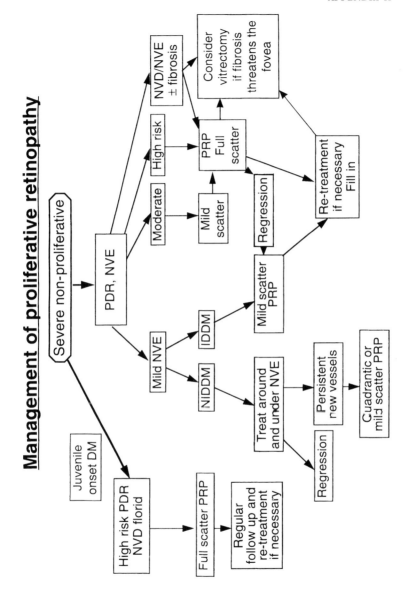

Combined macular oedema and proliferative retinopathy

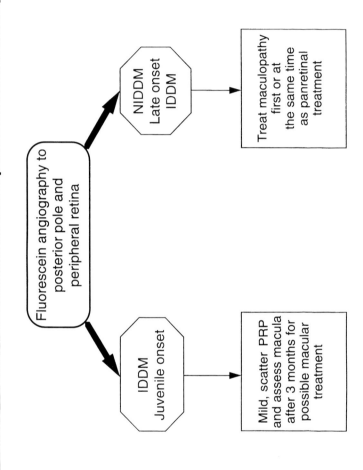

Fluorescein angiography to posterior pole and peripheral retina

IDDM Juvenile onset

Mild, scatter PRP and assess macula after 3 months for possible macular treatment

NIDDM Late onset IDDM

Treat maculopathy first or at the same time as panretinal treatment

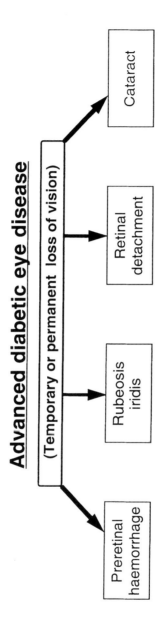

Advanced diabetic eye disease
(Temporary or permanent loss of vision)

Cataract

Retinal detachment

Rubeosis iridis

Preretinal haemorrhage

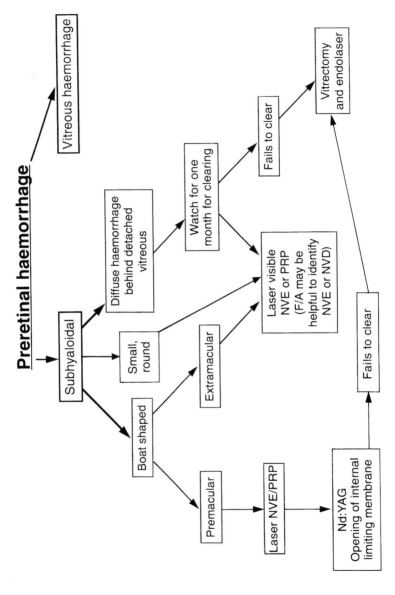

Vitreous haemorrhage

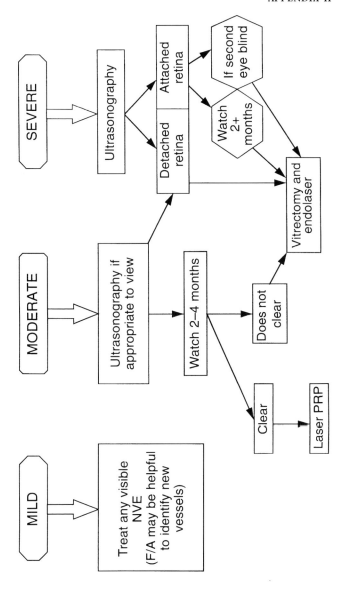

Diabetic rubeosis

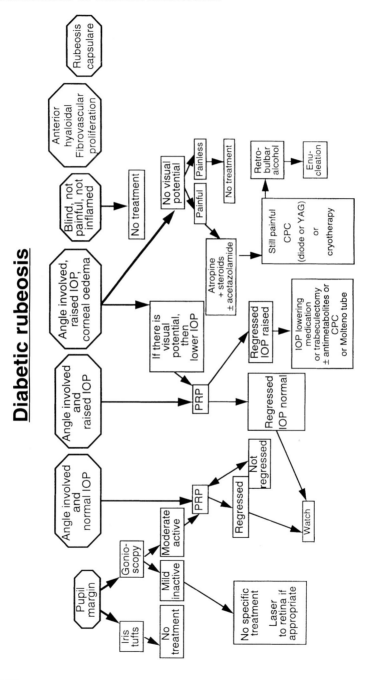

Anterior hyaloidal fibrovascular proliferation

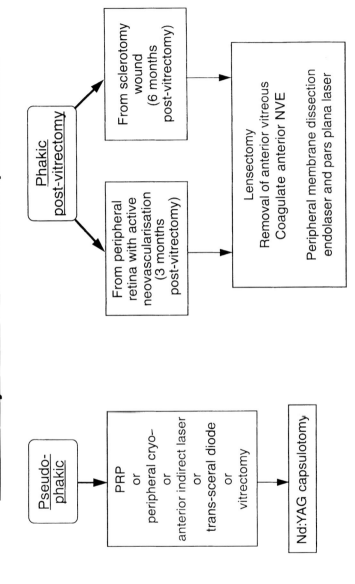

Phakic
post-vitrectomy

From sclerotomy wound
(6 months post-vitrectomy)

From peripheral retina with active neovascularisation
(3 months post-vitrectomy)

Lensectomy
Removal of anterior vitreous
Coagulate anterior NVE

Peripheral membrane dissection endolaser and pars plana laser

Pseudo-phakic

PRP
or
peripheral cryo–
or
anterior indirect laser
or
trans-sceral diode
or
vitrectomy

Nd:YAG capsulotomy

277

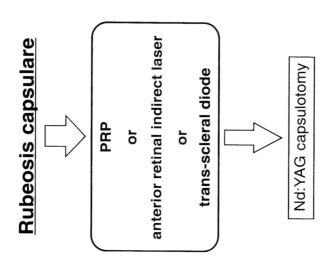

Rubeosis capsulare

PRP
or
anterior retinal indirect laser
or
trans-scleral diode

Nd:YAG capsulotomy

Diabetic retinal detachment

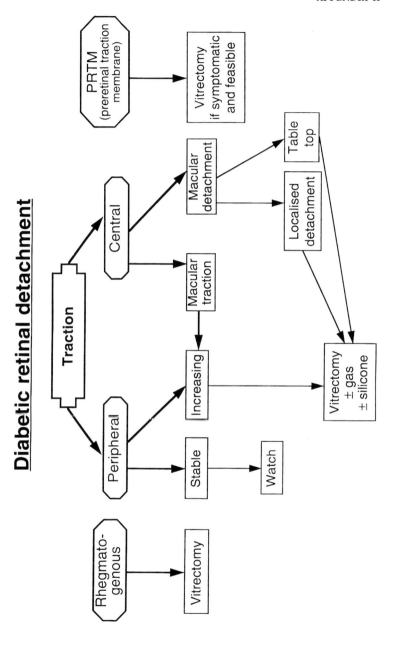

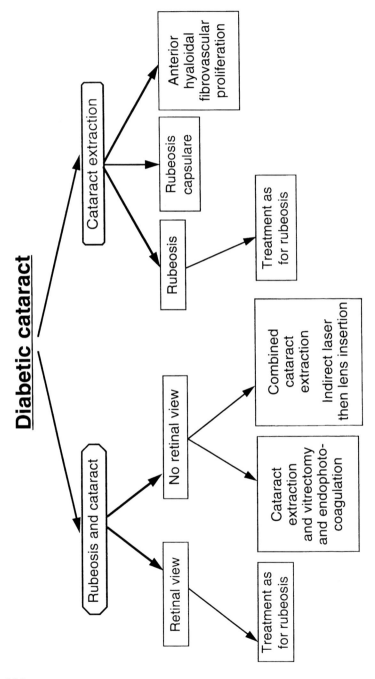

Diabetic cataract extraction ± capsular rupture

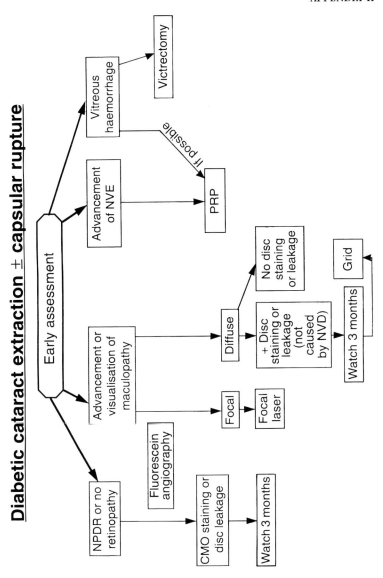

Further reading

Akiba J, Arzabe C, Trempe C. Posterior vitreous detachment and neovascularization in diabetic retinopathy. *Ophthalmology* 1990; **97**:889–91.

Ashton N. Neovascularization in ocular disease. *Trans Ophthalmol Soc* 1961;**81**:145–61.

Aylward GW, Pearson RV, Jagger JD, Hamilton AMP. Extensive argon laser photocoagulation in the treatment of proliferative diabetic retinopathy. *Br J Ophthalmol* 1989;**73**:196–201.

Benson WE. Cataract surgery and diabetic retinopathy. *Curr Opin Ophthalmol* 1992;**3**:396–400.

Berninger TA, Canning C, Strong N, Gunduz K, Arden GB. Using argon laser blue light reduces ophthalmologists' color contrast sensitivity. *Arch Ophthalmol* 1989;**107**:1453–8.

Brinchmann-Hansen O, Dahl-Jorgensen K, Sandvik L, Hanssen KF. Blood glucose concentrations and progression of diabetic retinopathy: the seven year results of the Oslo Study. *BMJ* 1992; **304**:19–22.

Buzney SM, McMeel JW, Field RA. Florid diabetic retinopathy: a role for pituitary ablation. In: Henkind P, ed, *Acta XXIV International Congress of Ophthalmology.* Philadelphia: Lippincott, 1983:788.

Chase HP, Garg SK, Marshall G. Cigarette smoking increases the risk of albuminuria among subjects with type I diabetes. *JAMA* 1991;**265**:614–17.

Diabetes Control and Complications Trial Research Group (DCCT). The effect of intensive treatment of diabetes on the development and progression of long-term complications in insulin-dependent diabetes mellitus. *N Engl J Med* 1993;**329**: 977–86.

Diabetic Retinopathy Study Research Group. Preliminary report on the effects of photocoagulation therapy. *Am J Ophthalmol* 1976;**81**:383–96.

Dodson PM, Gibson JM. Long term follow-up of and underlying medical conditions in patients with diabetic exudative maculopathy. *Eye* 1991;5:699–703.

Early Treatment Diabetic Retinopathy Study Group. *Ophthalmology* 1991;**98**(suppl 5):739–834.

Fankhauser F, van der Zypen E, Kwasniewska S, Rol P, England C. Transscleral cyclo photocoagulation using a neodymium: YAG laser. *Ophthal Surg* 1986;**17**:94–100.

Gabel VP, Birngruber R, Gunther-Koszka H, Puliafito CA. Nd: YAG laser photodisruption of hemorrhagic detachment of the internal limiting membrane. *Am J Ophthalmol* 1989;**107**:33–7.

Gabel VP, Lorenz B, Obana A, Vogel A, Birngruber R. Problems of clinical application of diode lasers. *Lasers Light Ophthalmol* 1992;**4**(3/4):157–63.

Grant M, Russel B, Fitzgerald C, Merimee J. Insulin like growth factors in vitreous. Studies in control and diabetes subjects with neovascularization. *Diabetes* 1986;**35**:416–20.

Grant M, Jerdan J, Merimee TJ. Insulin like growth factor I modulates endothelial cell chemotaxis. *J Clin Endocrin Metab* 1987;**65**:370–1.

Grant MB, Guay C, Marsh R. Insulin like growth factor I stimulates proliferation, migration, and plasminogen activator release by human retinal pigment epithelium cells. *Curr Eye Res* 1990;**9**: 323–35.

Green WR. Systemic disease with retinal involvement. In: Spenser WH, ed, *Ophthalmic pathology: an atlas and textbook*, 3rd edn. Philadelphia: WB Saunders, 1986:1034–210.

Heidenkummer HP, Mangouritsas G, Kampik A. Clinical application and results of Nd:YAG cyclocoagulation in refractory glaucoma. *Klin Monatsbl Augenheilkd* 1991;**198**:174–80.

Higgins PJ, Bunn HF. Kinetic analysis of the nonenzymatic glycosylation of hemoglobin. *J Biol Chem* 1981;**256**:5204–8.

Hiscott P, Cooling RJ, Rosen P, Garner A. The pathology of abortive neovascular outgrowths from the retina. *Graefes Arch Clin Exp Ophthalmol* 1992;**230**:531–6.

Janovic-Peterson L, Peterson CM. Diabetic retinopathy. *Clin Obstet Gynecol* 1991;**34**:516–25.

Kampik A, Ulbig M. Diabetic retinopathy. *Curr Opin Ophthalmol* 1990;**1**:161–6.

Khauli RB, Novick AC, Steinmuiller DR, *et al.* Comparison of renal transplantation and dialysis in rehabilitation of diabetic endstage renal disease patients. *Urology* 1986;**27**:521–5.

Klein BE, Klein A, Moss ES. Is aspirin usage associated with diabetic retinopathy? *Diabetes Care* 1987;**10**:600–3.

Klein BEK, Moss SE, Klein R. Is menarche associated with diabetic retinopathy? *Diabetes Care* 1990;**13**:1064.

Knowler WC, Bennet PH, Ballintine EJ. Increased incidence of retinopathy in diabetics with elevated blood pressure: a six-year follow-up study in Pima indians. *N Engl J Med* 1990;**302**:645–50.

Kostraba JN, Klein R, Dorman JS, *et al.* The epidemiology of diabetes complications. Study IV. Correlates of diabetic background and proliferative retinopathy. *Am J Epidemiol* 1991; **133**:381–91.

KROC Collaborative Study Group. Blood glucose control and the evolution of diabetic retinopathy and albuminuria. A preliminary multicenter trial. *N Engl J Med* 1984;**311**:365–72.

Lewis H, Abrams GW, Williams GA. Anterior hyaloidal fibrovascular proliferation after diabetic vitrectomy. *Am J Ophthalmol* 1987;**104**:607–13.

McHugh JDA, Marshall J, ffytche TJ, Hamilton AM, Raven A. Macular photocoagulation of human retina with a diode laser: a comparative histopathological study. *Lasers Light Ophthalmol* 1990;**3**:11–28.

Merimee TJ. A follow-up study of vascular disease in growth hormone deficient dwarfs with diabetes. *N Engl J Med* 1978; **298**:1217.

Merimee TJ. Diabetic retinopathy. A synthesis of perspectives. *N Engl J Med* 1990;**322**:978–83.

Miller JA, Gravallese E, Bunn HF. Nonenzymatic glycosylation of erythrocyte membrane proteins: relevance to diabetes. *J Clin Invest* 1980;**65**:896–901.

Moss SE, Klein R, Klein BE. Association of cigarette smoking with diabetic retinopathy. *Diabetes Care* 1991;**14**:119–26.

Moss SE, Klein R, Klein BEK. Alcohol consumption and the prevalence of diabetic retinopathy. *Ophthalmology* 1992;**99**: 926–32.

Olk RJ. Argon-green (514 nm) versus krypton red (647 nm) modified grid laser photocoagulation for diffuse diabetic macular edema. *Ophthalmology* 1990;**97**:1101–13.

Parving HH, Hommel E, Mathiesen E, *et al.* Prevalence of microalbuminuria, arterial hypertension, retinopathy, and nephropathy in diabetes mellitus. *BMJ* 1988;**296**:156–60.

Schatz H, Atienza D, McDonald HR, Johnson RN. Severe diabetic retinopathy after cataract surgery. *Am J Ophthalmol* 1994;**117**: 314–21.

Segato T, Midena E, Grigoletto F, *et al.* The epidemiology and prevalence of diabetic retinopathy in the Veneto region of North-East Italy. *Diabetic Med* 1991;**8**:11–16.

Skuta GL, Beeson CC, Higginbotham EJ, *et al.* Intraoperative mitomycin versus postoperative 5-fluorouracil in high-risk glaucoma filtering surgery. *Ophthalmology* 1992;**99**:438–44.

Sorbinil Retinopathy Trial Research Group. A randomized trial of sorbinil, an aldose reductase inhibitor, in diabetic retinopathy. *Arch Ophthalmol* 1990;**108**:1234–44.

Thompson JR, Du L, Rosenthal AL. Recent trends in the registration of blindness and partial sight in Leicestershire. *Br J Ophthalmol* 1989;**73**:95–9.

Ulbig MW, Kampik A, Landgraf R, Land W. The influence of combined pancreatic and renal transplantation on advanced diabetic retinopathy. *Transplant Proc* 1987;**19**:3554–6.

Ulbig MW, Kampik A, Thurau S, Landgraf R, Land W. Long-term follow-up of diabetic retinopathy up to 71 months (mean 38 months) after combined renal and pancreatic transplantation. *Graefes Arch Clin Exp Ophthalmol* 1991;**229**:242–5.

Ulbig MW, Hykin PG, Foss AJE, Schwartz SD, Hamilton AMP. Anterior hyaloidal fibrovascular proliferation following cataract surgery in diabetic eyes. *Am J Ophthalmol* 1993;**115**:321–6.

Ulbig MW, McHugh JDA, Hamilton AMP. Clinical comparison of semiconductor diode versus neodymium:YAG non-contact cyclo photocoagulation. *Br J Ophthalmol* 1995;**79**:569–74.

Ulbig MW, Arden GB, Hamilton AMP. Color contrast sensitivity and pattern electroretinographic findings after diode and argon laser photocoagulation in diabetic retinopathy. *Am J Ophthalmol* 1994;**117**:583–8.

Ulbig MW, McHugh JDA, McNaught AI, Hamilton AMP. Contact cyclo photocoagulation for refractory glaucoma with a diode laser. A pilot study. *German J Ophthalmol* 1994;**3**:212–15.

Ulbig MW, McHugh JDA, Hamilton AMP. Diode laser photocoagulation for diabetic macular oedema. *Br J Ophthalmol* 1995;**79**:318–21.

Wong HC, Sehmi KS, McLeod D. Abortive neovascular outgrowths discovered during vitrectomy for diabetic vitreous haemorrhage. *Graefes Arch Clin Exp Ophthalmol* 1989;**227**: 237–40.

Young RJ, McCulloch DK, Prescott RJ, Clarke BF. Alcohol: another risk factor for diabetic retinopathy. *BMJ* 1984;**288**: 1035–7.

Index